LIFE IN BETWEEN

Natalie Smith

This book is dedicated to anyone who has gone through the trauma of ulcerative colitis, whether you are a patient or a patient's loved one. You are not alone.

And to anyone who has written a book. It's harder than it looks, right?

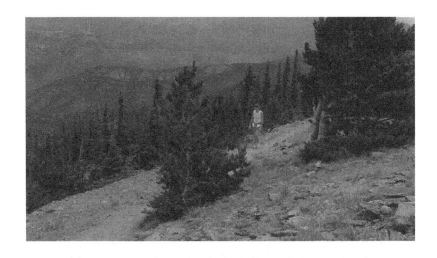

PREFACE

My name is Natalie and I'm a sibling recovering from the hurricane-force winds that Ulcerative Colitis (UC) stirs up. As your narrator for the next two hundred or so pages, I'm grateful you picked up this book, one that I never knew needed to be written until the dust finally settled for my family in mid-2017. When the "you need to write a book" lightbulb went off during a casual conversation with my older sister, Danielle, this story's heroine, I exclaimed that she should find time to make it happen. Lives would be changed, I argued. Hope would be restored. Yes, pen needed to be put to paper in order to inspire others in similar, very unfortunate shoes, to keep going in the aftermath of this unnatural disaster. Without hesitation, she said, "No, Nat. You should write it."

There were numerous moments in Danielle's journey, as you'll read, that I was present for and am able to describe as an eyewitness. For the earlier portion of this story, however, I was not living in the same city. Danielle was in New York State and I was 1,184 miles away in sunny Orlando, thus, I relied on my family to fill in the exact details. Over the course of many months, many Friday night dinner conversations, and many stolen moments in my office with my laptop, this labor of love came to fruition.

The stories included within these pages are at times harrowing, at times comical, but overall, very personal for all who lived through it (my family and I) and especially for Danielle who lived with this rotten disease. According to the Centers for Disease Control in 2015, 1.3% of adults in America reported being diagnosed with either UC or Crohn's disease. With UC, the "ulcerative" portion represents teeny weenie, itty bitty, little baby ulcers on the inside of one's colon, a.k.a. the large intestine. Those small ulcers are what causes blood to be present when you have a bowel movement. A lot of it. Scary amounts. And the "colitis" portion means inflammation of the colon. It's mad as hell and isn't going to take it anymore!

If you're lucky enough to be completely, blissfully unaware of this enigmatic disorder like I was for most of my life, here is my unscientific description: it's as if terrible, dreadful, and horrendous got together and created an inflammatory bowel disease. Sounds fabulous, right? And let's focus quickly on the word "bowel." It's not a word that invokes happy thoughts or a word most people want to use on any given day. It's an area of the body not frequently discussed at dinner parties or at the water cooler. Can you imagine if it was? Can you imagine having UC and having to discuss it more publicly?

"Hey Jeannie, heard your bowel is giving you lots of trouble today. Do you want to talk about the color of your stool? How's the consistency?"

"Bob, your bowel acting up again? Do you want to push back our 10:00 meeting? It's cool, everyone poops."

Nope. That doesn't happen. People are uncomfortable chatting about the nether region that dispenses excrement. Yet, we all have these parts. We all go to the bathroom, boring number one and the unsexy number two. For folks living with UC, however, they experience unpleasant symptoms that directly interfere with their daily lives with respect to going number two. And most of us existing around these people are completely unaware. These same folks, my favorite colon-fighting superheroes, are doing everything in their power to try to live as conventionally as possible. As if their rear end isn't raw with extraordinary pain for having gone to the bathroom an average of 10 times a day.

When I say "gone to the bathroom," that's a euphemism for what you can imagine as the worst diarrhea imaginable. Then there's weight loss, malnutrition, fevers, waking up in the middle of the night to go (some nights multiple times), stomach cramping, and the bonus -- as if all that wasn't enough, is a susceptibility to many other disorders thanks to a weakened immune system. Think more colds. More sore throats. And... jackpot! Sometimes other GI (gastrointestinal) issues like *Clostridium difficile* (a.k.a. *C. diff*, but more on that joy later) find their way into the mess of things. Not only do UC patients have to contend with one major GI illness, but sometimes it can be compounded into two.

Before I forget, I need to mention something important: UC is not something you catch from others and it cannot be relieved with a simple pill. It falls under the large umbrella of auto-immune diseases, an unattractive list of afflictions that include multiple sclerosis, celiac disease, rheumatoid arthritis, alopecia, and type 1 diabetes, just to name a handful. This means that your own body pulls the ultimate *Mean Girls* attack on itself and tries to wreak havoc. With UC or Crohn's, the unlucky location is your GI tract. I liken Crohn's to UC's even meaner first cousin. I say meaner because it is not limited to one section within the GI tract like UC. Crohn's can appear and do damage at any point along your food journey – the esophagus, the stomach, the small intestine, or the large intestine. It makes it a lot trickier to treat and can pop up in multiple spots with healthy tissues located in between diseased areas.

According to the Mayo Clinic, a known cause for UC has yet to be discovered. Initially, doctors hypothesized that a person's diet and stress factors were to blame for the inflammation. Now they believe those just simply magnify the disorder. They believe that heredity plays a greater role and there is a snafu in the body's immune system response.

(Side note - a wise editor of this book pointed out to me that SNAFU has roots as a military acronym. Did you know that? Reportedly, it stands for "Situation Normal: All F*@#$d Up." These diseases definitely fit that bill.)

It's possible that when trying to fight off a pesky virus or bacterium, something goes awry and the immune-fighting warriors we usually rely on opt for the Ethel and Julius Rosenburg turncoat approach. They start attacking our own good gut bacteria, setting the stage for UC.

Sounds fun right? I apologize for painting a depressing picture, but this is the real portrait in living a life with a colon that is hell-bent on self-destructing and taking down everyone around it. Most days, those of us on the outside feel helpless and those who drew the extremely unlucky UC straw are confined to the toilet or a bed. It isn't glamorous, it isn't wonderful, and it can persist for many years, as you'll see with Danielle's tale I'm about to share.

Along the way you'll meet the characters of our lives that played an integral role in helping my sister recover from the very dark lands to which UC catapulted her. At times you won't believe your eyes. She endured procedures, treatments, tubes in places tubes have no business being, long hospital stays, and even longer nights at home that you wouldn't wish upon your sworn enemy.

This is why I wanted to share her journey. Hope is real. Healing is real. Poop is also real. And so is recovery. Here's a story that marries these things in the best of ways.

Prayer, magical unicorns, rosary beads, whatever you believe and however you need to get there, having faith in the human spirit to transcend turmoil can create tangible effects. Enjoy.

CHAPTER 1

She lay there with her cheek pressed against the cream-colored rug while her one-year-old daughter May played around her. Danielle had shut the bedroom door, locking them in so that May couldn't find trouble out of her sight that needed attention. Danielle was not in good shape. And definitely not in any kind of shape to take care of her cherubic, gap-toothed blonde daughter that was relying on her for safety.

Danielle's thoughts were cloudy and disrupted by a fever so traumatic she would later describe it as one that caused pain to every cell in her body. She ached internally as she lay listless against the carpet. As the minutes ticked by in the morning hours of this Thursday in late September 2011, she wondered how long she'd have to exist in this state until her husband came home to take over. Could she make it or would her angry invader win? What had taken over her normally very healthy 33-year-old self?

As she trembled, she continued to believe that she was just a typical, run-down, young mom who contracted a bug.

"This is just the stomach flu. I'm just a tired mother with two small children, this will pass," she thought to herself.

From outside May's bedroom she heard the deep

voice of her father-in-law Gregg.

"Danielle? Are you home? May?" he called.

In a whisper, Danielle tried to alert Gregg of her whereabouts. Thankfully, their ranch-style home was not too spread out, and he eventually discovered Danielle laying there while his youngest granddaughter toddled around her mother with a smile and a giggle, protected by the bliss that shelters children in serious situations.

"Danielle, Bill called and asked me to come and take May home with me," Gregg said, hiding his shock and concern.

In a grateful twist of fate seven years earlier, Bill, her husband, and Danielle had moved back from Morgantown, West Virginia after college (Let's Go Mountaineers!) to their small hometown of Olean (Go Huskies!) in Western New York State and had unexpectedly landed two doors down from Bill's parents, Gregg and Rhonda.

Gregg and Rhonda are kind and supportive parents, the type you don't mind living next to because they grant you space but also are right there to help when you need their support or a cup of sugar. They both care deeply for their kids and grandkids and have always treated Danielle like a true member of their family. Gregg is a decorated Vietnam veteran receiving the distinguished Purple Heart, among other honors. He was wounded in battle and valiantly fought for our country at a time when he didn't have a choice. He is also the consummate jokester who taught all three of his children, Erica, Bill, and Gregory, an enviable wit. For example, if you were to strike up a conversation with Gregg at a party, it might go as such:

Gregg: "How about that henweigh?"

You: "I'm sorry, what's a henweigh?"

Gregg: "Eh, about six pounds."

Or you might be privileged to hear an alternative version. Insert the word "hamcost" or "cowsay." First-timers always get a good chuckle when they hear his punch line.

Rhonda is the sweet complement to her husband. She has strawberry blonde red hair and is very thoughtful and big-hearted; so much so that no matter what you put on your adult Christmas list each year, she (and Santa) will make it happen. In the past, Bill has asked for and received, a gorilla costume and a breathalyzer gun, because life is more fun if you have both of those in your closet.

At the time that Danielle was laying on the carpet, Rhonda worked full-time in Olean's city government building while Gregg was a retired master union pipe fitter who, thankfully, was home when Bill called. That was the second important call made that morning after it was understood that Danielle was in peril. The first came from our mother, Susan.

An hour prior, Susan, had come to pick up Danielle's oldest daughter, Lily, and take her to Sonshine Nursery school just down the road. Lily was three and had just started school. Normally on a Thursday in late September, Danielle wouldn't be home. Her sandy brown hair with golden highlights would be curled to frame her slender face and her makeup would be done almost effortlessly to accentuate her lovely brown eyes. She'd be wearing a posh outfit off the rack from Ann Taylor that formed perfectly to her size eight figure. And she would be standing at the head of the class teaching the young minds of Salamanca Middle School's eighth grade social studies students about the cause and effect of yellow journalism and the rise of muckrakers.

That wasn't the case on this day, however, because she had decided to take a second year off after May was born to stay at home with her kids. It was a decision that Bill and Danielle didn't take lightly. In fact, like many working moms, Danielle fretted over the choice for many months. Could they afford their home and their lifestyle on Bill's income alone? Would she be able to handle two kids under two? Deep down inside Danielle's belly, though, she knew that she would never regret an extra year with her girls and decided to delay going back until the following school year. In hindsight, the universe may have given her the nudge she needed to make the decision because she would need a great deal of that extra time to recover from what was to come.

This particular morning, where the story starts, Danielle had called Susan, a.k.a. "the big guns," to take Lily to school. On her first day of Sonshine a week earlier, shy little Lily clung to her mother's leg with toddler desperation. She held on with brute strength that one would not expect from a 35-pound preschool kiddo. Like many children her age, Lily did not appreciate the separation in the same way that stay-at-home mothers do when they are able to drop their kids off for a few hours (YAY!). Because of Lily's trepidation, Danielle enlisted the help of Gregg to take her the second day. The mission was not successful however when Gregg crumbled at the first sight of Lily's big, fat, alligator tears. That left the biggest ammo Danielle had, her own mother.

For as long as we've known our mom, she's had bangs, jet-black hair, and loves her Maybelline Brownish Black mascara and Cover Girl blush (always in the Peach hue). More importantly, I would describe her as a strong-willed Sicilian lady who wants nothing but to have her four children grow up to be happy and healthy. She is a typical mother in that sense but she has her quirks. She likes things the way she likes them and does things the way she wants them done.

For example, if she wants a dresser moved from one room to the next, she just does it – without fancy furniture movers, or help from anyone else. We tease her that she could toss furniture on her back and move it with the ease of ten men.

Susan tells you what she thinks and makes no excuses for it.

She is also extremely generous and wants the best for everyone in her circle.

"Do you need a new Yankee Candle for your bathroom? Here, take one of mine," she'd say.

"Did I hear you need new sneakers? Take this old gift card I have for the shoe store; I'll never use it," she'd ask as she dug for it in her purse.

She is also a task-oriented person, which, as a Registered Nurse (RN), suits her very well. She is an excellent nurse, and at that time back in 2011, had worked at the local hospital for almost 20 years.

When she had arrived to pick up Lily, she wasn't fully "ready" for her day to begin. And by that, I mean she did not have her makeup on and her hair was not done. Like most women, she didn't leave the house, with confidence, if those two tasks were not executed fully. However, she was running behind that day and decided to brave the potential nursery-school-mom glares and take Lily anyway.

To say she was stunned upon entering Danielle's house that Thursday morning is an understatement. She would have been less surprised had she been greeted with a breathalyzer-toting man in a gorilla suit. She was dumbfounded and scared, just upon laying eyes on Danielle. At first glance, she noticed Danielle's cheekbone protruding from her face because her cheeks were sunken so far inward. She was lying in the middle of the living room floor looking pale and gaunt.

After Bill had left for work at 8:00, Danielle had mustered up the effort to get Lily fed and dressed for school. But that was it. She could no longer keep on truckin'. She didn't pick up the dishes from breakfast, she didn't brush her hair, and she didn't do the multitude of other normal tasks she would have completed on a morning when she was well. All she could do was find a nice spot on the living room floor and lay there until our mom arrived to pick up Lily.

"Oh my God Danielle! Hang tight. I'm calling Bill and I will be back once I drop Lily off. We will get you taken care of."

Susan took Lily to school, ran home quickly to finish getting herself ready for the day, and then called Bill. She would later recollect that by calling Bill she was pulling the meddling mother-in-law card from her deck. But she was steadfast in her decision. Every mother-in-law has one and she knew this was her time to lay it out on the table.

"Bill, what the hell is going on? She looks awful and needs to get to the hospital right now!"

Though Bill is a tall fella, standing at a solid six feet, two inches, he is also an optimistic humorous guy. He was given the gift of eternal boyish good looks and soft blue eyes. His sandy blonde hair, always styled well, accents his all-American charm. But what sets Bill apart from the crowd is his ability to crack a joke out of thin air. He is not worrisome and generally has a sunny disposition. And although he would come to understand the severity of his wife's current state, he did not realize it as it was happening. Like Danielle, he wanted to attribute her symptoms to other things because that was the logical choice. It never occurred to either of them that a monstrous auto-immune disorder was behind the curtain slowly pulling the strings. He thought what she thought.

"She's just tired. She's overdoing it. She's a young mom."

Despite the overt signs present, he, being a supportive husband, was taking his cues from Danielle. Until this phone call with Susan, Bill believed she had come down with a bad case of the flu.

Little did he know...

CHAPTER 2

While commotion swirled around Danielle after Bill had rushed home to get her to the doctor, per Susan's order, Danielle reflected on what events led her to this moment. How could she have landed in such a scary state of despair? Sure, she liked traveling just as much as the next gal and there were still states left to visit on her bucket list but "I think I'd rather die than live another second like this" was not a locale for which she had ever fantasized about.

Let's flash back to the week before this moment and take a gander into what her life looked like:

Friday (6 days prior to her current position on the carpet)

One of the many benefits to living in a climate with cold winters and moderate summers are the perennial apple trees that allow for picking when September rolls around. Danielle and a cadre of playgroup moms decided to take their kids to a small apple picking spot in town. It was a delightful day and the kids enjoyed themselves running between the trees. But that is not what stuck out to Danielle as she analyzed Friday. She focused in on the fact that she had to change her clothes three separate times before leaving the house because she had an irritating fever and she was sweating through them all.

Why on earth would she have kept her plans that

day knowing she had a terrible fever? I asked the same head-slapping question. Even though she had perspired through three shirts prior to leaving, it was not a typical fever. It did not resemble the kind that comes with influenza. She did not have aches and only on occasion did she have the chills. She never had a sore throat or a runny nose. She just had a fever and increasingly worse diarrhea. So, she became best friends with the Motrin in her medicine cabinet and continued on with life. However, for anyone well versed in UC culture and its dos and don'ts, you know that one of the first things you discover about the disorder is that Motrin is on the banned list of drugs allowed. It helped her bring her fevers down, but it was not helping the festering ulcers building in her colon.

Despite the ups and downs she experienced while apple picking earlier in the day, Danielle and Bill had planned a fun night ahead. Bill had just received a substantial promotion at work, both in title and in salary, and his team members wanted to go out and celebrate with him. She had curled her hair and put on her best face but, internally, she was still battling with herself on what these symptoms could be.

By the end of the night, her bouncy curls had wilted and her hair clung to her sweaty face, again, thanks to her intermittent fevers. On the ride home, while the other people in the car were having a raucous good time (someone may or may not have been mooning passing cars), Danielle was shivering and shaking. She tried to crack a smile and support Bill and his accomplishments but the harder she fought to feel normal, the more unwell she felt.

Saturday

As the morning sun peeked into her room, Danielle knew she had to harness what little strength she had and get through the day as best as she could. She made it through apple picking, so she was optimistic she could will herself better. She pondered the prior Saturday (another seven days into the past) and realized not much had changed in a week. Actually, it had, but she did not want to admit it.

Bill had been participating in a summer golf league and that previous Saturday was their final tournament. For any stay-at-home mom that sentence translates to: "Congratulations! You get to play Cruise Ship Entertainment Director, housekeeper, and chef for not just five but six full days in a row!" And when your body is slowly failing, it makes it even more of a prize. She mustered the energy to get through lunch and dinner but had to throw the towel in and call Susan out of desperation.

"Mom, I feel really overwhelmed. I can't seem to get out of this funk. I'm just utterly exhausted."

For most people, a call like that is very hard to make. But she felt like she didn't have a choice. She wanted to give up. On both ends of the phone, the internal consensus was that she may be depressed. That could potentially explain the weight loss. And certainly, the energy depletion. Plus, she had small kids. Maybe it was postpartum they all surmised.

Part of the reason that they concluded it was not a life-threatening sickness and maybe just a mental health issue was that Danielle was not entirely honest with *both* my mom and our stepfather, Steve.

She wasn't dishonest either.

When she would discuss with my mom (a nurse) how she felt, she mentioned the occasional blood in her stools. Yet, when she talked with Steve (a doctor) about her physical state, she discussed the occasional abdominal discomfort and pain. And because neither my mom nor Steve thought that something was tremendously wrong, they never made the connection together that there were multiple symptoms actually occurring.

You might be wondering why a nurse and doctor could have overlooked these illness indicators but here's the reason for why that happened: they were looking for horses not zebras.

A common medical school adage that students are taught refers to the idea that when you figuratively hear hoofprints, you should look for something common and logical versus an outlier or a condition that's extremely rare. In other words, if you were walking down a road and heard hoofprints coming from behind you, when you turned around to see what was there, the odds of seeing a horse are much greater than the odds of seeing a zebra. With Danielle, she was young, she was otherwise healthy, she had just had a baby, and she was home all day with small children. It was not a stretch to think that she just needed more time and a boost to her mental wellness to get her over whatever hump she was stuck on.

Thus, ten minutes after she called them, Steve and our half-siblings Madison, who was 15 at the time, and Noah, who was 13, came to see if they could help. Madison and Noah watched Danielle's girls while Steve took Danielle down the street for a walk to see if he could lend an ear and provide the emotional support that she needed.

"Steve, I just want to be able to do my dishes. And I can't. I just don't have the energy," she whimpered.

She kept crying and he just listened.

Steve has a bald head and a salt and pepper colored beard. He has a big heart that matches his stature. He loves puzzles, politics, and has a new-found passion for gardening. He's also extremely smart. Aside from having the letters MD after his name with a focus in anesthesiology, Steve also has a PhD in Psychology. And a Master's of Great Life Advice from the world-renowned school of hard knocks. In fact, our stepmother Shayne was also blessed with the same honorary degree. We are extremely lucky to have both of them in our corner.

Steve came into our world just before Shayne, and although we love him dearly now, he was not accepted with open arms by our sardonic teenage selves. He was new and he wasn't our father. He was patient, though, and kind, and willing to wait for us both to come around. He was a child of divorce and had also endured a traumatic situation before marrying our mom. His first wife was in a horrific car accident just before their wedding and was left wheelchair-bound with the mental capacity of a small child. They were married anyway, as he tried to do the right and moral thing. Unfortunately, it didn't work out. I imagine that both events helped shape Steve into the extremely thoughtful step-parent he has become for both of us.

Stepping back even further in time, on the day of Danielle's high school graduation in 1996, my mom held a small gathering at our house by our pool, an in-ground pool that my dad had put in the summer before they split up. In the cement by the stairs, I wrote "Welcome to the Certo's" with my finger, a forever reminder of whose house it was initially. My mom and Steve gave Danielle a nice set of luggage to take with her out to Arizona for her big college move that was on the horizon. Upon opening the luggage, our beloved Gram, my mom's mother, pushed Danielle to go give Steve a hug. It was forced and awkward but yet it was a huge step forward for us. In retrospect, I'm sure Danielle was resentful in that moment, but it was a pivotal gesture that helped thaw the ice that existed.

With Shayne, it was a little easier to let her in. She was also a child of a divorce and had also gone through a divorce herself shortly before meeting my dad. She's a gorgeously positive person inside and out and was extremely gentle in meeting us. She was never pushy nor was she absent. I remember the first time I met her very clearly. I was 13 and went to dinner at the apartment where she and my dad lived. It was a third-floor walkup with amazing details and charm. It had high ceilings and the character of the old Victorian home that it was housed in. I can't remember what they made for dinner but they offered to invite my childhood best friend and next-door neighbor, Amy, to come along to make it an easier experience for me. I don't recall ever looking up at her face but mostly just staring at the floor.

It was a lot to process at that age but once that first meeting occurred, it became more comfortable to invite her into my world. She has blonde hair, great taste in makeup and perfume, and a luminous personality unlike most people. She's equally as fantastic as Steve and an incredible mom to our other half-siblings, Victoria and Andrea, who are both in their early twenties now.

Returning back to that one summer day, though, when Danielle was melancholy — Steve was just what Danielle needed. On their walk he was kind and nonjudgmental. He reiterated to her that he and my mom were always there and would lend a hand with whatever, whenever she needed it.

She remembered that pep talk on this current Saturday, the day after apple picking, when she held onto hope that maybe she needed to be more positive. Because she's a teacher and teachers are exemplary problem solvers, she attacked her potential self-diagnosed depression with a plan.

She thought to herself, "What if I just need to branch out in the community and be of service to others who need it? Maybe I could lend my talents for being creative with those who could also use a pick-me-up in their lives?"

Danielle had been taking Lily and May to our wonderful hometown library for afternoon crafts and really appreciated the way she felt once they left. The girls were happy to have used their hands to create something and Danielle could visibly see the joy it brought them. After some self-reflection and soul-searching, she decided to call our local soup kitchen to see if there could be a time for such an activity with their guests. She was excited to hear the enthusiasm on the other end of the phone when she pitched the initial idea. She even went as far as meeting with the manager at the site and even discussed a budget for the crafts she'd be teaching. Since it was September, she researched Halloween and Thanksgiving craft ideas and was looking forward to pulling herself out of the doldrums with which she was stuck.

Do doldrums include diarrhea, though?

Unfortunately for the soup kitchen, her grand ideas never came to fruition as you'll soon read. Her volunteer aspirations would be squelched by her uncooperative bowel. At the time, though, she could rationalize that if she was depressed, that would be the cause for her fatigue. What, then, could be causing the unrelenting bathroom trips?

"Despite never throwing up, maybe it is the stomach flu? That could be what's triggering the fevers and the unsettled stomach," she rationalized in her mind.

Regardless of the cause and her justifications for what was occurring, she was scheduled for her waitressing shift that night at Angees; a night that happened to be mandatory for all employees, part time and full time. It was "Parents Weekend" at St. Bonaventure University, our local college, and it was always incredibly busy. Thus, it was all hands-on deck and she needed to bring her best waitressing game with her when she punched in.

Because life is more fun with layers and layers of complexities, let's add one more ingredient to her pot before we continue. Even though things had started to turn south, at the beginning of the summer Danielle had decided to take on this moonlighting waitressing gig because she was no longer receiving her teaching salary. She still enjoyed (and deserved) an occasional stroll through Banana Republic so she landed as a waitress two nights a week at a local Italian restaurant, Angee's, that has been open for more than half a century. We started going there as kids with our dad who had come to know the owner quite well. And all through college she had donned an apron and had served folks, first at The Outback, and then at Kegler's in Morgantown (again, Go Mountaineers!). She knew her way around a kitchen and complaining customers. It was an easy job and worth the benefits. The best benefit was the free meal she could bring home each night she worked. Her favorite was always the steak and cheese sandwich on a crusty, Italian roll.

However good her intentions were, waitressing was just another drain on her deteriorating immune system. Many of the summer nights she worked, she was dashing around the restaurant for three to four hours solid. She would then get home late and had to turn around and get up early with the girls in the morning. When the weight started to come off at a hastened pace, Danielle attributed it to her extra daily steps fetching ketchup and merlot for the locals. She even made it a point to add broccoli and other dense, nutrient-rich foods, to her daily intake, thinking that she needed to add more vitamins and calories to her day and that would help her energy level, fingers crossed behind her back.

Back to Saturday: going into her shift she knew that either she'd have a wardrobe change either from her fevers or from her newly found superpower, fecal incontinence. She shared with one of the other waitresses that she may be "fighting off the flu" and, if in a pinch, she may need backup. The waitress was kind and thoughtful and told Danielle she had her back if needed.

[A brief post-COVID pause is in order here. It seems shocking that someone could have gone into work knowingly carrying a virus with them but in reality, Danielle knew

something was really and truly wrong, beyond a stomach bug. She secretly knew it wasn't the "flu" but the "flu" was an easily understood moniker for what could be brewing in her body. This was pre-COVID, when people weren't using words like, "contagious," "incubation period," and "transmission." As sordid as it may be in 2021, it was common for people to work through an illness up until March of 2020.]

Thankfully, adrenaline is a helpful hormone and it carried her through the long, arduous night and provided her a break from the toilet.

Sunday

Home, sweet home. When she woke, she handed Bill the grocery list as well as her parenting card. She was punching out from that job and planned to stay in bed all day long. For any mother reading this, you know what an excruciating task that is to complete. Whether you are physically out of commission or not, it's no easy feat to "be sick" while you are home with your family. But to have a fighting chance at overcoming "this flu" she knew that's what she needed to do: tag out and rest.

Monday

hooray with a lowercase "h." She felt better. She was by no means in the clear but she had regained some of her strength thanks to her temporary hiatus. She made it through the day and thought that when Bill came home from work, they could venture out on one of their nightly walks with the kids and their dog, Truman.

In thinking about this particular nightly walk, she remembered it being punctuated with a mid-way stop on a park bench because she was out of oomph. Her legs could no longer carry her so she had no choice but to tell

Bill she needed a rest.

"Do you mind if we stop here Bill? I'm sure it's probably all part of my recovery from the sickness I had over the weekend."

However, another nightly walk, now permanently etched in her brain from earlier in the season, should have clued her in that something was amiss. She did not make it to a restroom in time when she had the urge to go. Thankfully, she had some extra clothes with her and was able to trash the soiled stuff in the garbage can of a local pizza joint. Bill, being the comedian that he is, took it in stride and joked with Danielle about "the poor bastard who would have to take that trash out at the end of the night. I wouldn't want to be that guy!" He was trying to lighten the mood and make her feel less uncomfortable about what just occurred: while out for a stroll, she had pooped her pants... in front of her husband.

And while we're on the topic of exercise, the last run she went on before her fevers began left her feeling extremely discouraged. With each step she took her legs felt heavy, as if they were weighted down and her sneakers were superglued to the ground. She struggled to keep going and had to stop much sooner than she would have liked. She knew she was out of shape after being pregnant but this felt different. It felt like something was happening that she had no control over, which put an end to an activity that normally made her feel invigorated and proud.

Tuesday

Uncle.

Danielle woke up and decided to call her doctor.

Amazingly, she was able to get an appointment for that day but was not able to see her normal doctor. Instead, she was seen by two residents who may now be excellent doctors, but at the time were probably scared and nervous young adults trying not to screw up. They were not attuned to Danielle as a patient and most certainly did not understand the severity of her condition. They explained that her diarrhea could be caused from an awful germ known as *Listeria*, which can be found in spoiled food, and during that time, there was an outbreak of it from bad cantaloupes.

Yes, that was their possible diagnosis of her symptoms – rotten fruit induced flu. They sent her on her merry way with a stool sample kit so they could check for *Listeria*.

The voice that lives inside your belly that wards off bad decisions was speaking up and telling Danielle she needed to fess up to those around her. This wasn't the flu. It wasn't bad cantaloupes. Something was wrong and she was finally coming to grips with it. She was also startled to see the number on the scale. She was down 15 pounds from her normal weight. On her way home from the doctor's office, she stopped at the grocery store and bought a package of chocolate chip muffins and apple cider since the broccoli just wasn't cutting it. To heck with vitamins, she needed tasty calories and she needed them quick.

When she explained her plight and her appointment to my mom and Steve, they continued their supportive stance and told her that she could try Imodium for the diarrhea and that maybe, just maybe, it was an awful case of *Listeria*.

Wednesday

No improvement.

In fact, the energy she had on Monday was nowhere to be found. She called the doctor's office back and let them know she really felt bad. She explained that she actually felt worse.

"I completed the stool test but I don't believe this is *Listeria*. Is there something else I can do?"

They decided to get some blood work from her so she made her way to the lab with the hope of finding some answers.

Upon returning home while she waited for the results, she began to look back at the last year and connected the dots that had been floating around her all along. She realized that there was an obvious and chronologically-sound journey present that she would become best friends with, having not only lived it, but having to retell it numerous times to family and a multitude of medical professionals.

Her story started like all notable narratives and most fairytales do, with hemorrhoids.

"Once upon a time, long, long ago, there lived a beautiful princess in an old castle. This princess was extra special. She was blessed with a swollen vein in her rectum that causes pain, blood, and sometimes extra trips to the commode."

Can you handle all that excitement?

After giving birth to May in June of 2010, Danielle assumed she had a bad case of hemorrhoids, which is a typical side effect of pregnancy. Mothers have the privilege of pushing a very large object (a tiny human) out of a very small place and your prize is more discomfort and lots of creams. The nuisance associated with this common condition persisted, though, so she decided it would be prudent to mention it to her OBGYN doctor the summer before during her six-week post-partum check-up. The conversation should have gone like this:

"So, Danielle, how are you feeling? Are there any things you'd like to talk to me about?"

"Well, I experience a lot of blood when I go to the bathroom. My rear end is really sore and I'm in the bathroom quite a bit, which is not a normal routine for me. I sometimes worry I won't make it to the toilet and I often feel energy-depleted. By the end of the night, I'm kaput. And with two small kids at home, I can't afford to feel like this. I've increased my food intake and have tried to add in nutrient-rich foods to help but it doesn't seem to be working."

"Danielle that sounds serious and more than just hemorrhoids. I think we should send you for blood work and a consultation with a gastrointestinal doctor (GI). I will make a call and get you in to see one very soon. I'm so glad you are taking your health so seriously and making it a priority."

Unfortunately, that's not what happened. It should have. It could have.

But it didn't.

Danielle, like every strong woman walking this earth right now with a to-do list a mile long, believed that she was complaining and not living up to the tough standard that she witnessed as a child from her mother Susan, her grandmother Josephine, and her great-grandmother, Venezia Del Bianco.

Venezia, as a nineteen-year-old girl who spoke no English, boarded a steamer ship to cross the Atlantic and left the Old Country of Italy behind. All three were tough Italian broads who took it on the chin and kept going. Certainly, she could get through this, Danielle thought.

So, the conversation really went something like this:

"Danielle, how are you feeling? Are there any things you'd like to talk to me about?"

Think of what a mouse's voice would sound like if they could talk. And then take it down another octave for Danielle's reply.

"I'm feeling good. Well, there may be a smidge of blood when I go to the bathroom. Just a smidge…"

"It could be postpartum hemorrhoids?" she asked.

"Yes, that's it! It's hemorrhoids!" Danielle said feeling relieved the issue plaguing her was a simple one. "Sure, I'll use that cream! Yes, I'll reapply a few times a day! Thank you!"

Regrettably, her UC Spidey senses were not fully developed at that appointment, much to the dismay of everyone around her who would come to realize that this was a fork-in-the-road-moment of her story. If she had shared the serious details with her doctor, truthfully, the doctor may have recognized that UC was gearing up to rear its very ugly head and her symptoms should not be ignored. More tests would have likely been run and her progress monitored more closely. Instead, Danielle wanted so desperately to be normal and healthy again and clung to the idea hemorrhoids were to blame.

Things never got better, though.

Sigh.

By autumn of 2010, one year prior to when and where this story started, her symptoms were amplified. Someone had cranked up the volume and she began to get worried. She had endured the wrath of May's colic for the majority of the summer and now this was occurring. Hip, hip, hooray!

If you have never been blessed to hold the role of stay-at-home-mom-in-chief it's worth researching. Moms are fascinating in the best ways possible. Even with the comforts that we're all used to nowadays (iPhones, iPads, Amazon Prime, etc.) they are still a force to be marveled at and celebrated. With regard to how tough-as-nails UC survivors are, Danielle was a champion. At that time, she had to care for an infant, a toddler, a husband, and the very large German Shepard man-dog, Truman, who liked to eat TV remotes as a mid-morning snack.

A funny canine aside: A few years before Lily and May were born, Truman, a fine-looking dog with a palette for finer cuisine, smelled wonderful odors coming out of Danielle's crockpot. He decided, with assurance, that he was the better recipient of the meal Danielle had planned for that night's dinner, prime rib that had been simmering all day. He took it upon his four-legged self to pull the pot from out of the wall and off the counter. He emptied the expensive contents into his belly, and then dragged it into the living room onto their nice, lightly colored, tan rug. He then proceeded to lick the pot clean. Every. Last. Morsel. When he managed to get the pot off the counter (without the assistance of opposable thumbs, I'd like to point out), the pot fell to the ground so hard it damaged the brand-new tile floor. It had also caused quite the splatter of au jus on their kitchen wall. Being such a large dog, Truman could jump up on two legs and reach great heights. In fact, when Bill came home each night, Truman could jump up as if to lock in an embrace, and his paws were almost to Bill's shoulders. As I said earlier, Bill is tall guy. So, imagine a wall completely licked clean to about six feet — and then higher than that, lots and lots of meat juice speckles. Bravo, Truman!

But, back to the glory of being a mom who doesn't go off to work each day — as a baseline, she had to cook three meals a day, get up at night to feed May, do the loads and loads of laundry that come with having an infant, shop for groceries, entertain Truman to the lifestyle he was accustomed, and engage her kids in fun activities. Every single day. Rinse and repeat.

Now imagine the joys of that job and imagine that you have to go to the bathroom frequently and with urgency. In other words, having diarrhea five, six, even seven or more times a day. And before you can get to the toilet that you so desperately need to get to, you have to make sure your two danger-prone kiddos are taken care of and out of harm's way. May was a special risk because she was still very small.

All of these factors combined, caused Danielle to often have to bring May in to the bathroom with her, or leave the bathroom door open. Now picture the fact that she didn't always know when the urge would strike and sometimes, she was not prepared for it because it was all so new to her way of existing in the world. Think of the stress this might cause her – now think of the stress it would cause you. An uncomfortable thought, right?

By November of 2010, five months into her new-found problem, our mother and Steve were looking to move across town. Danielle and the girls went with them to tour the new property they were hoping to buy. It was a spacious, beautiful, Tudor-style home with a lot of stairs and a considerable amount of square feet. They did eventually purchase it but it stuck out in the timeline Danielle was mentally reviewing as a moment when she recognized the literal and proverbial shit was getting real. Her colon was not playing anymore. She realized quickly that an accident could be impending when touring the new home at this open house, and she was more than ex-tremely grateful that there was a stash of toilet paper in the bathroom she commandeered.

"Phew. Thank you, sweet baby Jesus. That was a close one!" she thought to herself.

That's when Danielle, a former parochial school kid who grew up to be Catholic in-name-only, began to pray. She prayed to God Almighty harder than she had ever prayed before.

"Dear God. Please, please make this go away. Please make this go away. I'll be good. I'll go to church. I'll give to the needy. I'll stop taking the last of the orange juice. I won't secretly cut anyone in line again at the grocery just so I can get home sooner. I won't just pretend to listen to Bill when he talks too long about work. I need to get through our trip to Italy and Natalie's bridal shower and wedding. Please help me do that."

She repeated that prayer every night for the rest

of the winter, trying to mentally will herself to get better and cause whatever this was to retreat and stay in hibernation for eternity because Danielle was looking ahead. In 2009, she and her bosom buddy and best teacher-friend Alexis, started an International Club for their students, and in mid-April of 2011 they were taking their maiden voyage to Italy. She and 30 students, including chaperones and family members of hers, Bill, myself, our sister Madison, and Bill's parents, were all going to board an Al Italia flight across the Atlantic for what she hoped would be ten joyful and gelato-ful days. Not only was she in charge of making sure the logistics of the trip went smoothly for everyone involved, she also had the added pressure of taking 30 children to a foreign country and have them all return home safe and unscathed.

To add to the incredibly large plate she was balancing, at the end of May, just a month after the big trip, my then fiancé, Mike, and I were getting married, and she was my Matron of Honor. Therefore, she was also responsible for the execution of my bridal events. Thankfully, we were well matched: I was a very low-key bride who just wanted everyone to have a swell time, and Danielle was a master party planner, even before Pinterest was a thing. The only downside for her was the timeline. We were set to fly home from Rome on a Thursday night and the shower was to be held just two days later. She knew that having to run to the bathroom during the trip to Italy or during the wedding festivities would very much be a curse and not a blessing.

She pored over every detail of the trip and spent a great amount of time preparing for my special day. She envisioned a gorgeous spring shower over brunch, held at a mountaintop restaurant. To keep the fun of the day going, she wrote a clever poem for me to read at the end of the party that would clue me in on the bachelorette event we were to embark on that evening. Instead of penis-shaped cookies and scantily clad men, she knew I'd enjoy a Moroccan cooking class followed by a very fun and interesting belly dancing lesson. Her ideas were focused on me and what I'd prefer, and did not center on anything else. Selflessness says a lot about a person, especially one who was living in a toilet hell at the time the party planning was happening.

She needed for the God of Toilet Paper to hear her pleas and make some changes. She did not need this diarrhea distraction.

By January of 2011, things pivoted in the right direction. Hallelujah! After the holidays had come and gone, life seemed rosier and required a lot less Charmin. She was able to once again live her life without fear or hemorrhoid cream (because at this point, she still believed that it was hemorrhoids ailing her). Spring trickled in, the birds chirped, the sun returned to Western New York, and so had her smile. She was eternally grateful that her problem had taken a hike, without a lick of an explanation or reasoning.

By the time we needed to pack our suitcases for Italy in April of 2011, things had really turned the corner. The trip was molto bene (really great)! The students and chaperones loved it. The pizza was phenomenal, and the pinot grigio was cheap. We left our homeland with a newfound appreciation for our family members who began their lives there. It put us both in great spirits as we relished in the fun of my bridal shower and bachelorette party, which were both delightful occasions. I can also say the same about my wedding. She was able to appreciate each celebration to the fullest. Her "hemorrhoids" were kept at bay and she felt that life had returned to being enjoyable.

Until "they" decided to come back.

One morning in June, a month after my wedding, she was down at the end of her sleepy, dead-end street with her daughters, enjoying the warm weather. If you live in the Great White North that is Western New York and the weather is even remotely agreeable, you are compelled to be outside soaking it in. So, there they were, outside, feeling happy when suddenly Danielle's internal organs fired off a flare that let her know trouble was ahead and was approaching quickly.

Mayday! Mayday!

Danielle sprang from her feet and grabbed Lily and May by their hands. Poor little May, who was just about one, didn't want to leave her sunny spot. Like all good toddlers, she assumed the world revolved around her and was not about to move. The harder Danielle tried, the more May resisted and in the Big Battle at the End of Their Street, May was triumphant and Danielle's colon was not. Accident number one in what would become a hefty list of unfortunate fecal events. UC: 1, Danielle: 0.

Later that day, Danielle was outside watering her flowers when her neighbor stopped to chat.

"Gosh it really seemed like the girls, especially May, did not want to listen this morning," the neighbor stated.

Danielle grinned and thought to herself, "Lady, if you only knew why I was starting to lose my cool and why poor May had a DEFCON 1 meltdown! I didn't want them to go home nor did they want to. I needed them to move their feet though so I wouldn't defecate in my shorts. And guess what? I did!"

Yet, she chose the much politer and more neighborly comment instead, "Oh, I know. I really needed to get them home though."

The various signs were present that something was wrong, but as we move back to the Thursday in September of 2011 when she was prostrate to the ground, she still couldn't make sense of what was really happening.

This was what had brought her here: a baby, and then hemorrhoids, diarrhea, and then accidents, a depletion of energy, and then fevers. Mighty, mighty fevers that could go for days. This one, though, the one she had now in the present day of this retelling, was unlike any other. Her effort was valiant but despite it all, she was anemic and headed into a scary, septic state. Her opponent was so strong that even powerhouse, cruciferous vegetables like broccoli, and sugary confections like chocolate chip muffins, cannot conquer.

After Bill picked up Danielle, they started their journey for answers at her PCP's office. They had called ahead of time and alerted them. Without approval, they were on their way. On the walk to the doctor's office door, Bill had to basically carry his wife into the building because she was too weak to walk the short distance across the parking lot. Her head hung low and she was frail and feeble, a shadow of her normal self.

They saw the same two residents who hypothesized her affliction was *Listeria* initially and were again unsure of the correct path to take. They rationalized that they needed another round of data on Danielle before they could fully process her condition. They sent her across the street to our small-town hospital for more blood work and a CT scan of her abdomen.

It took about an hour for Danielle to have her blood drawn and for her to receive the scan of her belly. While she waited for the next direction and plan of action, Danielle, despite her despair and festering fever, advocated for herself. She used a new muscle she would learn to flex at various points along the way.

"Bill, I cannot go home like this. I'm afraid they are going to send me home to wait and I won't go. You cannot take me home. Something is really wrong."

If sending her home was to be part of the plan, we'll never know, because fate intervened in the form of febricity, a fancy word for fever. (I was afraid you'd become "fever" fatigued by the end of this story so I wanted to change it up. Variety is the spice of life after all.)

Keep reading and just for kicks keep a tally at how many times it's used to describe her. If you are over the age of 21 and were to take a shot for every time it's mentioned, you might even develop a temporary case of UC after the amount of alcohol you will consume.

This particular fever that came on in the hospital was a doozy. Danielle could feel it come on and does not remember much other than moaning like a wild animal caught in a rusty trap. It was a fiery feeling that came from deep within her. It caused the moaning and uncontrollable convulsing, all while she was still in the lab waiting room. Luckily, across the hall was a kind woman that Danielle had known for some time. She was the pre-anesthesia nurse and knew Danielle through our stepfather (since he was an Anesthesiologist who worked there at that time) but also because her son had gone to high school with Danielle. She dove into helping as if she was a triage nurse. She got Danielle a wheelchair, a toasty warm blanket, and gave her some Ibuprofen from her own purse because as a nurse and mom, she could see how terribly Danielle was suffering. This nurse, along with a lab tech, made the right decision by telling Bill they needed to head for the emergency room ASAP. Something scary was happening and they did not have time to waste.

A moonlighting PCP who practiced locally was assigned to Danielle's case in the ER — thank you to the higher power involved in allowing that intervention.

We have come to love and appreciate this doctor, and he now sees our entire family. On that day, though, he was just a good doctor, one who could hear the fright and desperation in Danielle's voice and wanted to do something about it. Her hellish fever made a second appearance while they waited in an ER bay for her results to come back. During this time, she was given fluids to help ease her strife temporarily while the doctor analyzed her most recent lab work.

For help in understanding how quickly she became gravely ill and how that lab work helped save her life, here is a quick tutorial (in case you can't remember from biology class) on what the following items measure and represent.

White blood cells (WBCs) are important because they fight off infections.

Red blood cells (RBCs) are equally important because they carry oxygen throughout the body.

Hemoglobin (HGB) and hematocrit (HCT) are tied together and often shortened to "H&H." They are significant to measure because they capture the amount of blood cells in one's body.

Now that you are basically a phlebotomist, here is a sampling of Danielle's blood work from back-to-back days.

On Wednesday, at 5:20 in the afternoon, when she was sent to get it drawn after she declared that it couldn't be *Listeria*, this is how it looked:

WBC: **6.6** (the normal range is 4.0 – 10.5 K/uL) = A normal reading.

RBC: **3.51** (the normal range is 4.20 – 5.40 M/uL) = A lower reading, but not scary low.

HGB: **11.1** (the normal range is 12.5 – 16.0 g/dL) = A lower reading, but not scary low.

HCT: **32.0** (the normal range is 37.0 – 47.0 %) = A lower reading, but not scary low.

Ultimately, the doctors reviewed it, my mom and Steve looked at it, and they all agreed it was not remarkable. It did not signify any major reason to worry.

Yet.

On Thursday, when she gave blood at the hospital at 12:22 in the afternoon, amidst her raging fever, she was still hovering at fairly normal(ish) levels.

WBC: **5.0** (the normal range is 4.0 – 10.5 K/uL) = A normal reading.

RBC: **3.71** (the normal range is 4.20 – 5.40 M/uL) = A lower reading, but not scary low.

HGB: **11.6** (the normal range is 12.5 – 16.0 g/dL) = A lower reading, but not scary low.

HCT: **33.9** (the normal range is 37.0 – 47.0 %) = A lower reading, but not scary low.

Given how acutely sick she was, though, the doctors decided that Danielle was not going home. She was immediately admitted to the ICU for treatment and her proverbial ball of medical issues started to roll. They were not aware of the lurking UC but they wondered if she was becoming septic, a diagnosis no one wants to receive.

Sepsis is both a doctor's nightmare and a sure-fire way to land a vacation in the hospital. It is caused by the body's inappropriate reaction to an infection. It occurs when chemicals are released into the bloodstream as a defense mechanism against a microorganism. It can cause damaging inflammation and ultimately, organ failure. When symptoms such as confusion, increased respiratory rate, and low blood pressure come on, a patient may have less than a day before the body really begins damaging itself. According to the National Institutes of Health, sepsis is one of the leading causes of disease-related deaths in hospitals. Further, according to the CDC, one in three patients who die in a hospital have sepsis. If an undiagnosed septic patient is sent home, tomorrow is never guaranteed.

Had Danielle gone on another day toughing it out at home, she would not have been able to "tough" it out even one more day.

Once Danielle was in a room in the ICU, about eight hours later, her blood was drawn again.

WBC: **2.7** (the normal range is 4.0 – 10.5 K/uL) = Bad.

RBC: **2.72** (the normal range is 4.20 – 5.40 M/uL) = Bad.

HGB: **8.4** (the normal range is 12.5 – 16.0 g/dL) = Bad.

HCT: **24.7** (the normal range is 37.0 – 47.0 %) = You guessed it — bad.

Her newest blood work revealed a very alarming picture. In eight short hours, her body had waged war, militarizing itself against an unknown enemy. A drop in her H&H levels that quickly hinted at one thing: active bleeding. In addition to her lab work, her vital signs showed that sepsis had now taken over a body that was already malnourished and anemic.

Around this time, my mom came to relieve Bill who went home to help his parents with the girls. She was about to set foot in Danielle's new home away from home and was told by the ICU nurse to wait outside. Given the circumstances, that was understandable, but it was not a relief for my mom. She wanted to be in there watching exactly what was happening to her oldest daughter who might not make it through the night. As a nurse, though, my mom knew the importance of helping a gravely ill patient without the added distraction of a distraught family member nearby.

While my mom impatiently paced in front of the door, Danielle thought she'd try a cool new party trick – fainting every minute or so. The nurse was trying to check her vitals and hook her up to various IVs, but Danielle's septic-ridden body was not cooperating. It was as if she was a snake being made to sit up straight. She repeatedly fell back into the bed vertebrae by vertebrae, time after time.

Simultaneously while she was receiving immediate treatment (and passing out), we, her family, began to make plans for how to care for Lily and May and to provide support for her and Bill. Mike and I were still living in Orlando at the time and, ironically, we had been planning on coming home that very weekend. We had back-to-back weddings to attend in the area and were going to be home for about ten days. Once she was admitted, I called the airline that same night and was able to bump up my flight from Saturday morning to the first flight out on Friday. Our small town is about an hour and fifteen minutes south of Buffalo and the nearest airfield so I needed someone to pick me up from the airport. I was extremely anxious and wanted more than anything to be teleported back home so I could be on the front lines helping. I couldn't make time speed up fast enough to get there. So, I did what a twenty-something girl does in this situation. I called the guy who was best-suited for the job; the guy who you call for hardware questions and anything car-related, my dad, Hank.

A quick word on our *other* quirky parent. We are fortunate to have two parents with novel idiosyncrasies that make them special, or as Danielle and I like to say, "Unique." Like Susan, Hank is unmatched. He's fifty percent Sicilian and fifty percent Polish - a stubborn combination of genes. However, his genes also blessed him with natural good looks. He stands at just under six feet with dark brown hair, olive skin, blue eyes, and striking facial features that make him a handsome gentleman. He has a voracious appetite for reading and an ear for classic rock music played really, really loud. His desire to play music extremely loud *always* seemed to occur when he would drop us off at school, work, or a friend's house.

Thanks Dad!

He, like my mom, is also incredibly generous. He's one hell of a cook and bread maker and was a third-generation partner in our family's beer distribution business, Certo Brothers, along with his siblings and cousins. Although he would have excelled in college (just sit and watch Jeopardy with him), he made the decision to go directly into the family business, which is where he stayed for the entirety of his career. Our family sold the company in early 2020, after having been in business for more than a century. It serviced the Buffalo and Niagara Falls areas as well as the area where we grew up, which is a pretty large territory to cover. He learned the art of respectful patronage and superior customer service from his father who had learned it from his father as well. As one might think, in his heyday, Hank enjoyed stopping by his customers' establishments to check on his draft beer systems and to buy other patrons a beer if they were drinking his product. Because of the large swath of land Certo Brothers encompassed, it meant he had a lot of customers. He was also a member of all the animal clubs: The Elks, The Moose Lodge, The Eagles Club, The Kitty Cat Club, etc. I'm kidding about the Kitty Cat Club but if there had been one and they were a customer, Hank would be a member. Now, it's customary for members of these lodges to stop by daily and "sign the book." It may seem silly to you and me, but to members, signing the daily book is part of the membership draw. It puts you in a daily drawing to win money and if you don't "sign the book," you can't win. Capisce?

So, if you're still with me, the relevance of Hank's book signing proclivity plays a role in Danielle's first night in the ICU and my trip home. He was in the ICU room with my sister when I called.

And my mother.

My parents had been divorced for many years at that point but it's fair to say, at that stage in their evolution as co-parents, they were not holding hands in prayer over Danielle. Times have changed quite a bit since then though and they get along great in present day.

"Dad, I moved my flight up and instead of arriving on Saturday with Mike, I'm taking the 6:00 flight tomorrow morning and will be in Buffalo around 9:00. Can you pick me up at the airport, please?"

That seems logical and understandable, right?

"Sure. I'd be happy to. But I have to make a stop and sign a book on my way up to get you so I may be thirty minutes late."

The flustered, red-faced "my parents are so annoying" feeling that you get when you're thirteen and your dad drops you off at middle school with "When the Levy Breaks," by Led Zeppelin, playing at full volume, started to awaken itself deep down in my stomach.

"But Dad I don't want to wait at the airport when I could be driving home to see Danielle. I can see if Mike's parents can come and pick me up."

"That's silly. I'll be there. I just might be late."

"I don't want to be late. I just want to get there!" I screamed.

That frustrated feeling fully awakened and was operating at maximum capacity. Meanwhile, my mom, and, to some degree, Danielle, despite the severity of the situation, began to smirk and giggle under their breath. They could hear my voice rise in protest as my insistent father tried to convince me that "signing the book" would not impact my timetable and I just needed to relax.

"Relax?! You're not listening to me!" I objected.

His comments were incendiary, and I thought I might explode in our downtown Orlando second-floor apartment. Eventually he relented, which I can now see was probably his plan all along. Sometimes he likes to argue for the sake of arguing and I fell right into it. Hook, line, and "book signing" sinker.

Danielle's eyes were closed throughout this argument but as he began to yell over me, she stopped being amused by it and shot my mom a look that communicated her need for it to stop.

"Henry, knock it off. She's trying to rest," my mom said.

As I was about to hang up, I asked if he could put the phone up to Danielle's ear.

"Danielle, I know you are fighting for your life right now, but if you die and leave me to deal with our crazy parents, so help me God, I will fly up to heaven and bring you right back down here. Do you understand me?"

Through the phone I could tell Danielle wanted to laugh but didn't have the energy. I was half kidding and half serious. She couldn't leave me to deal with both of them on my own. I told her I would see her tomorrow. Neither of us knew how long of a night she'd have ahead of her.

Danielle was utterly exhausted and not allowed to eat or drink anything while they were determining the cause of her sickness in case surgery was required. She hoped that she'd be able to close her eyes and wake up in the morning to some answers.

My mom and dad both went home to try and get some sleep. As a parent now myself, I cannot imagine the fear of leaving my child, adult or toddler, in an ICU bed not knowing just yet what was causing her to be so seriously ill but being made aware that it was touch and go.

If you ask Steve about this night, you will assuredly receive a guilt-ridden answer. His senses as a physician, and as a parent, were telling him he should sleep in the chair near her bed. He believed that if anything sudden arose, as a physician, he would be there as a proxy since she was so weak. Danielle being the consummate caretaker that she is, told him to go home and get some rest because she was hoping to do the same. She was also aware that if Steve stuck around, he'd have the displeasure of having to see her relieve herself in a bedpan. From her point of view, because she was so sick, he would have really only been helpful by assisting her to the bathroom when she needed to go. However, because of her septic state, getting out of bed to go was not an option so she had to rely on the bedpan. And although they are really close, having Steve around when the nurse came to clean it was a step-parenting bridge too far.

Another pattern you'll notice throughout these pages are the clear instances of Murphy's Law: if anything can go wrong, it will. In Danielle's case, if it was possible for things to go wrong, bad, south, haywire, sideways, it would, could, and did. Thus, on that first night in the hospital, Danielle did not slumber peacefully and dream of the shopping trip she would take to Banana Republic (and J.Crew!) once she was well. Instead, her nurse woke her to let her know she'd need a blood transfusion. Remember her hemoglobin and hematocrit levels from earlier? Because they had dropped so low in such a short amount of time, the intensivist (ICU doc) on call felt she needed blood and it couldn't wait until daylight.

The next issue they wanted to tackle was determining the cause for the shortness of breath they observed. In order to get a clearer picture of what they were dealing with, they decided it would be prudent to do a chest x-ray in the wee hours of the night. The two plausible possibilities for the abnormal breathing included: an excess of fluid building up in her lungs and pneumonia.

For a young person such as Danielle, being pumped full of fluid would not normally create an issue. For an extremely malnourished person such as Danielle in her current state, it was problematic. Her blood lacked the protein that draws in water, and keeps it, in her red blood cells. This was an involuntary byproduct of the poor nutrition she inadvertently was receiving thanks to the inconspicuous warlord that is ulcerative colitis. In essence, her cells were not holding in water, or fluid, because they didn't have enough protein to contain it. They simply weren't strong enough. Thus, the fluid was collecting elsewhere, in possible spots such as the lungs, an area of the body where fluid is not welcome.

They needed to also rule out pneumonia because she presented with some basic pneumonia symptoms: high fever, elevated white blood cell count, and now, a poor breathing pattern.

Too weak to travel on her own down to the x-ray department, they wheeled in a very large machine and snagged the images at her bedside. Thankfully, she did not adopt either malady. But just to be safe, they decided to give her Lasix, which is a diuretic medicine that made her have to pee, all the damn time. Because of her delicate condition, she also had to pee in a bedpan (oh the horror!), for the rest of the night.

When Danielle looks back on this night, her memory is not of the urine she sat in, or the blood they gave her, or the fact that she hadn't eaten in days. It was the tremendous feeling of thirst. A desperate thirst that seemed to consume her thoughts. Because she had been feverish for so many hours and because they were now giving her medicine to remove fluid from her body, she was dehydrated at a level most people cannot fathom. She was only allowed to chew on ice chips which were satiating but not enough to quench her intense desire for a tall glass of water.

So, she hatched a plan.

She was going to let the ice chips sit on her tray and melt so that it would feel like she was actually drinking something. The seconds ticked by and after what she would describe as thirty agonizing minutes, there was a sizeable puddle in her cup, along with a few ice chips remaining.

Hooray!

Success!

She reached for her cup and in her shakiness the lone ice chips rushed out first and startled her. The water she had so desperately longed for ran down her cheek onto her gown.

Dehydrated defeat.

The nurse on duty brought her more ice chips and Danielle waited once more.

She would also recall this night and the nurse who took care of her by remembering the sight of the nurse's shoes. Danielle looked down at the nurse's sneakers and wondered if they were comfortable. Because Danielle needed a great deal of care and attention, the nurse had been running laps all night long. Like an adult in her seventies and a supremely caring person, Danielle, who was in no shape to worry about someone else, was in fact worrying about someone else's arch support.

When the morning came the kind ER doctor who had admitted her, along with the intensivist, decided that she needed a colonoscopy test to determine if there was a colorectal disease at play. I have the fortune of not being old enough yet to have undergone a colonoscopy test myself, and up until this point, neither had Danielle. But for anyone of you who have, you understand that there is a preparation process that has to occur before they go searching around your colon so they can get a clear picture. For healthy folks, a delicious cocktail of MiraLAX must be consumed a day ahead of time that forces the body to rid itself of all the stool hanging out in the large intestine. For someone like Danielle, that wasn't an option. She didn't have time on her side nor was she well enough to get the drink down. They had to go with plan B: warm water enemas.

When you hear warm water enema you might initially think of something calming and relaxing. "Warm water" has an innately positive connotation. It's the third word, though, "enema," that mucks it up. The day nurse appeared before Danielle with a gallon of warm water, a tube, a bedside commode, and instructions that they were going to have to force this warm water into Danielle's rectum. She would then have to try and hold it for as long as possible before evacuating whatever she could, in the commode, next to a complete stranger.

This process would be horrible for anyone with a

healthy rear-end. But for someone with UC who has a raw, sore, infected one, it was astronomically painful (check out the first colonoscopy series of images and you'll understand what Danielle was working with). The nurse was empathetic and thoughtful and used the curtain in Danielle's room to create a makeshift divider that she'd jump behind every time Danielle had to evacuate so that there was some shred of privacy. She had to force water down the tube eighteen excruciating times. By the nineteenth time, Danielle vomited from the pain. Her body seized and she threw up out of pure misery.

At that point, the compassionate nurse exclaimed, "You poor baby. We have more water left but I'm making the decision that this is enough." Having said that, the nurse began to tear up out of sympathy. Her understanding of how agonizing this was for Danielle went beyond the nurse/patient relationship and touched her deeply on a human level.

Thankfully, Danielle was heavily sedated for the colonoscopy which revealed a red, oozy mess in her colon. It was confirmed on October 1, 2011 that she was in fact an ulcerative colitis patient and this would be with her for the rest of her life. That was the bad news. The good news was that someone much smarter than us in a lab somewhere had developed medication to help UC patients manage their symptoms and get them to hopefully retreat into remission. And the better news was that there was more than one smart person working on this who had developed a range of medicinal options. They started Danielle on a widely successful drug and were able to get her stable enough that she could leave her spa-like vacation in the ICU and head over to a normal hospital room.

This seemed like a great step in the right direction.

Now that she knew what had been ailing her, Danielle was relieved from the inside out. What she had been experiencing had a name. Lots of people experience the same thing. She wasn't just getting old and tired! She just needed to educate herself on what would become her new normal. She needed to know how to take care of herself in a way that would keep her symptoms at bay and afford her a sense of normalcy that she hadn't experienced in months.

One of the first consultations she received before getting the green light to high tail it out of there was to see a dietitian. And not just any dietitian, but my best friend's mother, Mary, who'd been practicing for decades. She was (and is) extremely experienced, wonderful to speak to, and the right person for Danielle to have in her corner.

She gave Danielle a myriad of things to try and provided her with a lot of information Danielle did not know. For example, if she were still dealing with a "flare up," she would need to avoid dairy completely. She also taught her how to add in true calorie and nutrient-rich foods and that if Danielle cooked food in a cast iron skillet, she would get some of that iron that she desperately needed. Also, she told Danielle that our bodies absorb nutrients from tomatoes if they are cooked together with a protein and eaten at the same time. Who knew?

Armed with a new education in healthy eating for those with UC, all she needed to get through were a couple more nights of medicated enemas and she was okay to be released.

The theme running throughout this narrative regarding Danielle's advocacy for herself made an appearance on one of her last nights in the hospital. It was time for her nightly enema and she was assigned a male night nurse who was set to help her with that job.

Let me explain, in case you've never had the pleasure and joy of a nightly enema, what that entails. A squirt bottle is filled with a medicated solution and that bottle is then carefully placed up the rectum and then squeezed until the contents are completely emptied in your rear end. Then you are asked to squeeze your cheeks together for as long as you possibly can before you evacuate said contents. At first Danielle could only do it for a matter of seconds. Toward the end of her stay, she could hold it for almost a minute. Practice makes perfect in the butt cheek Olympics - enema round.

For some reason, though, Danielle did not feel comfortable with this man as her enema companion given what they had to do. She reluctantly spoke up despite making a small wave by doing so and was given a female nurse. She didn't think about him again until months later when his name was in the local paper. That same night nurse had a penchant for pornographic images involving minors and was thankfully caught and put into jail. Creepy characters: 0. Danielle's intuition: 1.

While Danielle was recuperating, we as her family worked hard on the outside taking care of the life she abruptly left so that when she transitioned back home, it would be easy. After eight long days away from the familiarity of her own house, Danielle was released. We had the girls make signs, we bought flowers and balloons, and had dinner waiting. Although I had reservations about all of us waiting in her house for her arrival, she remembers it not as intrusive or overwhelming but as warm, comforting, and healing; knowing that she had a family willing to lift her up when she needed it.

CHAPTER 3

October turned to November and as the first Thanksgiving after her diagnosis came and went, we were all very thankful that Danielle was still with us. When something shakes your world, your perspective changes and you realize the gravity of the phrase "life and death situation." That is what happened for me anyway. I was 28 years old and had never been touched that close by mortality. I was completely content to not experience those emotions again, ever. At least not until I was really old with chin whiskers and cataracts. Until then, I wanted homeostasis.

Gratefully, I was able to maintain my warm Floridian homeostasis until late January of 2012. At that time Mike and I had been following up with his mother on a daily basis with regard to Mike's grandfather, Richard. A two-time war veteran and life-long Crohn's and shingles sufferer (as if one of those ailments wasn't enough to take on in a lifetime), he was unfortunately now succumbing to cancer and was not going to make it much longer. We were getting travel plans in place knowing that the day was going to come soon and we'd have to fly back home for the services.

I was not, however, expecting the first in a series of upsetting calls from my mother who stated, "it was back."

"What's back? IHOP's unending plate of pancakes?

The McRib sandwich?" I joked.

"Natalie, knock it off. Your sister is having fevers again and has become sick very quickly. She doesn't have UC symptoms, though, so we don't know what's going on."

My mom is not one to mince words and she's not one to stay calm. Her brain, like most mother brains, goes to a dark place almost immediately. Maybe it's to brace oneself for the incoming disaster? Maybe to fully prepare for the ominous events that could unfurl? If this is any indication of her demeanor and her naturally high level of tolerable adrenaline, she never misses *Twister, Jaws,* or *Poltergeist* when they are replayed on TV. My mom was worried and did not want to let Danielle know just how much. So, she called me and we tried to analyze what could be going on.

Although I have never earned a degree in anything related to medicine, my mom and I fumbled to try and retrace the last few months for Danielle to come up with a possible diagnosis that did not involve any words that remotely sounded like "ulcerative" and "colitis."

Was she just overly tired? Had she not fully recovered from before and had come down with something else, like the swine flu? Could it be the financial stress she and Bill were now enduring due to the medical bills that accrued during her eight lavish days in the hospital back in October? That could certainly send any normal, healthy person into a state of panic and account for body temperature fluctuations.

Danielle and Bill worked hard for their money and they were compensated well. However, they were not millionaires with a flowering money tree in their backyard. Apple trees, yes. Money trees, not so much. They, like most red-blooded Americans, did not expect nor have a contingency fund to cover the unexpected bills that were now before them. Danielle racked up a hefty bill, as one can imagine, with all of her healthcare interventions. They owed about $6,000 in actual bills needing to be paid – the total before insurance would kick in per her deductible. She owed for every provider she saw, every test she had to take, and every blanket she touched. Good health is important and it doesn't come cheap.

The frustrating part of the hospital bills she accrued was the timing — Danielle and her family had been covered under her school's insurance plan, a great plan, before she extended her maternity leave. But because she had opted to take off another full year, she lost those benefits and had to switch to being covered by Bill's plan, with far less attractive options. Overall, it would prove to be more costly. They were going from a filet mignon to a cube steak and as a result, were going to be out of pocket for a lot of dollars and a lot of cents. Plus, this was happening on only one income.

When she was well enough to join the land of the living back in November, when she was recuperating, she and Bill sat at her dining room table after the kids had gone to bed and itemized each bill to come up with a plan and a budget. They knew they couldn't tackle each bill all at once so they painstakingly called each provider and asked to be put on a payment plan that was realistic based on their finances. In some cases, it meant only sending in $5 or $10 per month just to show a good faith effort. Some kind souls in various billing departments even agreed to lower her amount owed given their dedication to making payments. Yay for humanity! However, it was still a monumental undertaking and ate up a sizeable portion of their monthly expenditures.

As January wore on, she was getting worse. She had once again lost the joie de vivre that she typically had in her voice. She is an overtly positive person with an optimistic, sunny outlook on the world she inhabits. But now, given her constant shivers and lousy quality of life, she had let dark clouds float in and we all watched in dismay as she was sliding backwards.

Here's how it progressed.

Danielle had been feeling good since the fall, post-hospital stay. Not good with a big "G," but still, good was better than having 18 bags of warm water thrust into your rectum by a stranger. With each passing week she was slowly regaining her strength, adding pounds, and building back her appetite. She was also extremely appreciative to be starting a new year with new health and a plan for what was now her new normal. As the frigid January began melt to away, though, she started to feel a little funny. Something seemed off but she couldn't put her finger on the cause. At first, her body responded like always, feverishly. "Feverish" would become my sister's adjective du jour for even more days to come.

Yet, she had no other symptoms. No runny nose, no cough, no tightening in her chest, and most importantly, she had no UC issues. She just came down with a fever one night after feeling not quite right for about a week. And that first night fever spawned other fevers that appeared throughout the day. After a full week of fevers, she was very ill, no longer good with even a lowercase "g."

Danielle's constant fever was now high and seemingly not taking a hike anytime soon.

My mom and I were at a loss for what could be happening. We spoke every day during the last week of January and each time she gave me the update, it seemed that Danielle's condition was worsening.

Danielle began to panic as well and finally pulled the trigger on getting herself to the ER one cold Thursday night. Bill took her after work, and unfortunately, she was a conundrum to the caregivers she saw. They tested her, drew her blood, and could not come up with a concrete diagnosis. They suggested she go home and contact her GI doctor in the morning because they concluded it could only be UC. She was mentally and physically depleted and unsure of what was happening.

Again.

By morning the fever was so bad she knew she needed to get into the bathtub to bring it down. When she stepped her toes in the tub, she started to cry. To sob would be a more accurate descriptor. A sob that embodied fear ("what is happening to me?"), disappointment ("I thought I checked off the 'being admitted into the hospital' box for the year"), and sadness ("sad for my kids, for Bill, and for my family"). While the tears fell into the warm tub, she worried she'd lose yet another week of her life to illness. Yet she promptly realized she had to pull it together and get Bill.

She was covered in a bright red rash from head to toe.

Before they could process what might be happening, their house phone rang and Bill answered. It was

Danielle's PCP, who had received her blood work from the ER overnight.

"Bill, you need to get Danielle to the hospital ASAP. Her white blood count is very low. We may need to have the oncology/hematology doctor examine her."

When Mike and I woke up on that same Friday morning to a cell phone vibrating, I assumed it was my mom calling me with a negative update on Danielle. I was correct in the bad news we were given; however, it wasn't my mom on the other line, it was Mike's. Sadly, his grandfather had made his way to heaven in the early hours of that morning, surrounded by all of his seven children. She was letting us know that we needed to fly home for the upcoming funeral. While we weren't surprised, it was still a sad morning as we packed, arranged for a pet sitter to come watch our dog, Hudson, and booked our flights.

As I tossed the last few items into my suitcase, my phone rang and this time it *was* my mother. She was barely able to speak. Distraught and frightened, she struggled to get the words out.

"Danielle is worse...PAUSE...They are calling in an oncology doctor...PAUSE... She's covered in a rash from head to toe...PAUSE... They think it is her blood...PAUSE... Oh my God, Natalie, what does this mean?" Now she was the one sobbing.

The hairs on my neck stood up and I got the chills. How could this be?

"Slow down, Mom. Maybe they are being abundantly cautious? She had no other symptoms until recently. We are hopping on the next flight to Buffalo, though, so I'll be there later this afternoon. Keep me posted and try not to get ahead of yourself. I'm sure it's nothing to worry about."

I lied like Pinocchio. I'm surprised she couldn't see my nose growing all the way from Florida.

Of course, it had to be something! In my eyes, doctors don't pull in an oncologist for a weird rash. Something must have told them to look in that direction. Lymphoma, leukemia? Terrible, awful thoughts rushed through my head. And although I hadn't dealt with it firsthand at that time, I had heard of the horrors my mother and my grandmother had witnessed with the loss of my grandfather in the late 1970s.

Phillip Catanese, my mother's father, was an attractive Sicilian man with a full head of dark hair and olive skin. He was a WWII veteran and stood a solid six feet and weighed about 180 pounds on a good day. I've always thought he resembled Robert DeNiro in the pictures I was shown as a child. He was beloved by his family, especially my Gram, and was taken out of this world too soon. At the age of 54, he was diagnosed with lymphoma, cancer of the lymph nodes. The Cleveland Clinic made the finding in April of 1976 and by the first week of October of that same year, he was laid to rest. Quick and extremely painful. My mom did not speak about him much when we were growing up because it was just too hard for her. As she grew older, the memories of him came more readily and they came with a smile. But the words "cancer" and "oncologist" were not part of a vocabulary she accessed. I could sense that her mind immediately flashed back to wearing bell bottoms and the *entire* year after he died when my Gram wore black — 365 days in a row of black ensembles. I knew she was worrying that Danielle could be facing the same fate.

When we hung up, I allowed myself to break down in tears before pulling myself together and heading for the Orlando airport. I am not a fan of flying. I could talk in front of 300 strangers but boarding an airplane makes my palms sweaty and my heart race. But on that flight home, I remember being overcome with sadness more than my normal fear response. We were not going home for a wedding, or a surprise party, or a holiday celebration. We were going home to a funeral and the unknown abyss of Danielle's sudden illness.

I distinctly remember looking around the plane and watching the happy families enjoying their fresh sun tans and Mickey Mouse ears as they headed home from a trip to Disney World. I remember feeling that our current situation on that plane was like a movie scene. Just hours earlier we had woken up to a normal day. Yet, after one phone call we were then throwing our stuff in a suitcase and running to the airport with heavy hearts. Mike and I didn't say much on the trip but kept checking our watches and our phones for updates while we flew up the Eastern Seaboard.

We landed in Buffalo, drove the painfully long ride to Olean, and parted ways. Mike headed to his parent's home to be with his grieving family while I found my way to Danielle's hospital room. I stepped onto the elevator and breathed in an all too familiar smell. Hospitals have such a particular scent, don't they? Weren't we just here a few months ago I wondered to myself? How could we be back so soon? I reached her room and took a deep breath in the hall before going in. I knew I would need to brace myself for what I would see once I entered.

Danielle would not have won a beauty contest and she would not have wanted to take a selfie. She was in rough shape. In fact, when I arrived, she didn't really even seem to register what was going on. Her sandy brown hair was flat against her head and her face was extremely rosy from the rash. It looked as if she had hiked up a volcano on the surface of the sun and then collapsed into bed. She shook and shivered, yet again, but tried to crack a smile when she saw me. My mom and step-dad were there as well and provided an update on the situation. They were still waiting for the oncologist/hematologist (blood doctor) to come and she was coming down from Buffalo. Although it was dinner time when I got there, the doctor would not arrive for quite some time which left us all to ruminate with scary cancer-like thoughts.

We received a break in the awful narrative of what was unfolding when the GI doctor, who was on call, stopped in to provide his feedback. He did not have any helpful conclusions, though. He went over her history with my mom answering most of the questions. They discussed the medicine that Danielle was currently taking. My mom mentioned that Danielle was forced to switch her daily UC medicine from the name brand, Asacol, to a generic counterpart in a different drug family, the sulfa family, back in November.

And here's why: a sad and extremely frustrating part of her narrative involves money. Remember the $6,000 they owed in hospital bills? Keep that in the back of your head as you read the following paragraph.

Just before the holidays Danielle visited her doctor to talk about other options with regard to her daily medications. Although they absolutely loved spending

$702 each month on an Asacol prescription, they thought there might be something else that was more affordable.

The first time Bill went to fill her prescriptions after exiting the hospital in October, the pharmacist told him the total due was a staggering $1,200 - $702 for the prescriptions that would be monthly, plus a few others she had to have immediately following her hospital stay.

Shocking, right? A one with three digits after it.

Doesn't that make you want to throw up to think about?

Or growl.

It makes me want to growl even to this day!

How is it possible that normal people are able to, as expected, magically generate money each month to that degree? And how is it possible that had they been under her insurance plan, the name brand medicine that was working, Asacol, would be much cheaper? Makes you want to throw up, growl *and* bang your head against the wall. Once she hit $6,000 for their deductible, the medicine would be covered but they had to hit that number first. So, they paid out of pocket until another visit with her doctor when he decided, per her request, to switch her to something much cheaper. Thus, the sulfas.

What my mom didn't realize in her report to the GI doctor on call, and what Danielle was too sick to communicate, was the fact that although Danielle was prescribed the sulfa medication back in November, she hadn't started taking them until January. Steve's brother, an internist in Buffalo, happened to have had some Asacol samples in his office and very kindly sent them down to Danielle to use. So, for an extra 45 days, she was getting the medicine that really seemed to work, and not using the sulfa drugs like everyone thought. According to her doctor's notes, though, based on the date the sulfas were prescribed to her, she had started the sulfas months prior to her current state. This is an important note in understanding how, once again, it took some detective work to identify what was truly going on with her.

The GI doctor took in everything my mom had to say and said it could be the UC. However, she was not symptomatic. Had she become septic from something else? Perhaps. They needed to do more tests to try and uncover what was at the root of this visit. I offered to sleep in the empty bed next to my sister so they could go home and get some rest while we waited for the oncologist to arrive. Danielle was so ill she didn't need much help or assistance. She slept, and shivered, and slept some more while I laid there and tried to fall asleep. If you have ever been unfortunate enough to stay overnight in a hospital, you know it's not a place of calm or respite. There are monitors going off in rooms nearby, nurses coming in to check vital signs every few hours, and doors opening and closing all around you. A constant reminder that health is important and when you don't have it, nothing else matters.

A little before 11:00 at night the oncologist finally arrived. She had reviewed Danielle's blood work and could safely say that cancer was not the cause. She also eased our worries that the only reason she was invited into the fold was the possibility of a blood disease but she did not think that was occurring, either. Her care team should have led with that when they mentioned needing her as a consult because until she made that pertinently clear, we were living in a world filled with worst-case scenarios.

On one hand, her news allowed us all to take a deep breath.

On the other hand, we were still left wondering.

When the sun peered through the hospital shades the next morning, our minds were still in motion trying to come up with the cause for Danielle's affliction. She was not any better and the rash was still fire engine red.

Nevertheless, it was not long before Danielle's favorite doctor swooped in to save the day. Remember how she met her PCP doctor in the ER when she was in there the very first time, back in October, and how he had run her blood work just to be safe, only to discover the raging UC war in her body? He put the pieces of her current puzzle together and realized that Danielle's problem could be solved if she just stopped taking her new, much cheaper, daily sulfa medication.

Because...she was having an adverse reaction to the sulfa!

In being able to speak to Danielle directly once she was more alert, he uncovered the fact that she hadn't been taking it since November and realized that she fit the bill for someone who was reacting to this particular medicine.

Hot damn, that was it.

A quick, very non-scientific Google search will tell you that the most common symptoms of a sulfa reaction are rashes and low blood counts, among other things.

Check and check.

In looking at her bloodwork again, it's apparent that the medicine started to negatively affect her immediately. When Danielle went for a normal follow up on January 7th, before her adverse reaction really took shape, her WBC (white blood count) level was already lower than what it should have been. In case you've forgotten already, in a healthy person, it would have registered between 4.5 – 11. Danielle's measurement was 3.6.

However, on the day of her admittance to the hospital, January 24th, it reached its nadir at a shockingly low level 1.3. Had she contracted another disease or virus, her body would have been ill prepared to fight it off appropriately, because, as I mentioned before, our WBCs are the front-line defenders of our immune response. Because of her extremely weakened state, and in order to protect her from other microorganisms, she was immediately placed in reverse isolation. Every time anyone entered her room, they had to wear a gown, a mask, and booties on their feet so as not to introduce any new pathogens into the space.

Her platelet level was also directly affected by the sulfa. On January 7th, her platelet count of 190 was within the normal range of 150-400. By the 24th, though, it had dropped down to 100.3 and dipped even lower to 74.1 on the 25th. The issues that can arise from having a low platelet count, or blood clotting mechanism, include increased bruising, fatigue, and the obvious one, the inability for your body to clot if you have a cut or laceration. The sulfa medicine was ravaging her body and she had no idea.

To add insult to the awfully painful injury Danielle was experiencing, my mother had urged her to make sure she was taking her medicine, even as she headed into the hospital the day before. If only they knew what was really occurring inside of her body with each dose.

An incredibly ill person is portrayed in her doctor's notes from the Saturday morning after her arrival:

REVIEW OF SYSTEMS: Not possible as the patient is pretty sick and somewhat groggy because she just received a dose of Dilaudid. She also has a headache.

PHYSICAL EXAMINATION: The patient is quite groggy. She is somnolent but arousable but falls right back to sleep.

VITAL SIGNS: Temperature this morning was 103.

SKIN: The patient has a diffuse maculopapular rash which is severe on her face and upper torso.

Translation: Danielle was not lucid, covered in an off-putting rash, suffered from a headache, and was still experiencing a high fever. It was after this assessment though that the adverse reaction was realized. Time needed to take its course before the medicine would be fully out of her system and her blood levels would find their way back to normal. She was given a steroid to help the process along and thankfully, that's all it took. Father Time needed to get in there and move the hours into days.

After five long ones, she regained enough of her strength and was given permission to be discharged. We welcomed her home just like we had three months prior, with signs, flowers, and relief-worn faces. It felt like we ran a marathon relay as a family and we finally reached the finish line. The best and worst feeling all wrapped into one sentiment, "Welcome home Danielle!"

CHAPTER 4

Winter in Western New York State, as mentioned before, is not a place where you go to cheer up. Don't get me wrong, fall and summer are gorgeous seasons around here and that's enough to keep us all going throughout the rest of the year. Oh, and we have the ultimate underdogs to cheer for, the Bills and Sabres (Let's Go Buffalo!). But for Danielle and Bill, they had the daunting task of once again trying to figure out how her super fun sulfa allergy would affect their already depleted monthly budget. They faced new hospital bills and the $702 per month Asacol prescription they wanted so desperately to get away from having. Thankfully she was given some samples to start her off. They then did their best to come up with a plan on Bill's salary and her weekly tips from waitressing until she could get back to work in September.

But let's stop here for a second folks, and recognize all the people who unwillingly have bought a ticket for this boat ride. The boat in which you hope to never find yourself aboard. A Noah's Arc full of people whose lives depend on a medication, or treatment, or procedure that will save their lives, yet it's ridiculously expensive and they can't afford it. Some go bankrupt, some choose a less effective option, some lean on their family, and some just figure it out. Danielle and Bill fell into the latter category and did what they had to do until September came around and Danielle could join her school's plan again.

Any guesses as to what she'd have to pay for her Asacol on her school's filet mignon plan?

A whopping $20.

That's it.

A difference of $682. But who's counting? Maybe not famous actors, sports stars, or millionaires. They are probably not counting with the same trepidation and dread that the greater population of us mere mortals would. However, Danielle would become a hometown celebrity for a brief minute in the spring of 2015, a bright and shiny spot that we all look back on with fondness.

I should also mention that in April of 2014 Mike and I made the decision to uproot our lives in Orlando and move ourselves, along with our one-year-old daughter, Sadie, back home so she could grow up surrounded by her family. It was more of a blessing than we could have imagined with regard to Danielle's health journey because it meant that we could be by her side for the tumultuous years that we didn't know were still ahead.

Back to the happiness of 2015, though. Danielle had remained healthy and strong throughout the prior three years and was able to afford her Asacol each month without selling her plasma, or soul, to attain it. Lily and May were now both in school and life seemed peachy until one day in early May 2015. During a quick lunch break in her room with her teaching partner-in-crime, Alexis, the school's superintendent interrupted them mid-bite to request Danielle's presence in his office. Though the tone in his voice was calm and somewhat excited, Danielle was alarmed because it was broadcast to everyone in the school. A similar instance occurred the week before, and it gave her and her fellow co-workers a good scare.

Six days prior to her lunchtime disruption, she had been in the middle of teaching a remedial class that consisted of only three students when she heard shrieking in the hallway. It was loud, unnerving, and increased in volume as time wore on. Before she could check out the situation, a shelter-in-place code was broadcasted across the school's loud speaker system. It was an alert that mandated everyone to find a room or stay in the one they were currently in until the situation resolved itself in the hallway. In this case, the unfolding and unsettling situation was directly outside of Danielle's room. She paused and could very clearly hear two young females screaming horrific cries.

"You're hurting me!"

"You're slicing me!"

"You're raping me!"

Accompanying the two young girls were two school officials trying to manage the situation as best as they could despite the heightened emotions swirling around them. At one point someone yelled that there was a knife and one of the girls was unwillingly wrestled to the floor. The contentious shelter-in-place situation lasted about 25 minutes before it de-escalated and the code was called off. Although Danielle and some of her co-workers were not directly involved, they still bore witness to the horrific ordeal and it impacted them for days after. They internalized the guttural screams they heard coming from the young girls and the fear written on their faces.

So, when the superintendent came on the school's

all-call PA system a week later, Danielle started to quietly cry out of fear that another, probably worse, incident was occurring. Their superintendent very rarely used the PA system and this was the second time in two weeks.

"Please excuse the interruption across the entire Junior-Senior and Seneca School campus. I would like Mrs. Eaton to come to the main office immediately."

The panic was written all over Danielle's face.

"This is good Danielle. I promise!" Alexis quickly assured her.

They abandoned their lunches, Danielle wiped away her tears, and they headed for the school's main office. But before Danielle exited her room, she was met by her closest colleagues who were all beaming with smiles waiting to escort her down the hall. She wanted to know what was going on but they held her off and told her she had to be patient. They were filled with pure jubilation and Danielle could see it. She started to worry less but the adrenaline then started to course through her body and she felt as if her knees were going to buckle.

When they reached the main office, the office staff started to clap for her in unison. When she reached the superintendent, he had an infectious grin on his face while he delivered some wonderful news.

"Danielle, you are making a difference and getting through to these kids. I received a call from the Live! With Kelly (Ripa) and Michael (Strahan) show. You have been nominated for their national Teacher of the Year search. Students and their parents wrote in on your behalf and they would like to include you in their group of 12 finalists."

Shock and awe took over as Danielle was overcome with gratitude. She was at a loss for words to describe her feelings. Check out the photo and her dumbfounded expression and the look of a true life-changing surprise.

She did know about the contest because I had also nominated her and had given her my submission letter simply to put a smile on her face. I've entered many contests and written many letters in my day and it's extremely rare to be contacted back. Neither of us ever thought that it would, and could, reach this level but we shouldn't have been so naïve. We should have taken into consideration the number of students whose lives had been positively impacted by Danielle during her tenure as a teacher. Her impact was so great that students and parents were also moved to take time out of their lives and share their feelings with a popular TV morning show in New York City. Because of that, we saw how strong a group of well-meaning folks can be.

The superintendent continued on to say that the show's producers had contacted him over email a few weeks prior and that the very next day her picture was going to be on TV. Kelly and Michael would read each finalist's name and that the national voting period would then begin. If she was selected after the 24-hour voting window as one of the final two teachers, she would get to visit the studio and be there live when they read the winning name.

She fought back happy tears and went back to her classroom. She picked up her phone, let the floodgates open, and began calling our family to share the excitement. I worked from home at the time, was nine months pregnant, and was scared to see her name on my phone in the middle of a workday. She's not on her cell phone much at all and is very professional about it not being around her while she teaches, a fact that drives our mother nuts, so much so that if she has a question throughout the day, she texts or calls Alexis to get to her. Knowing that, I feared the worst. I was further saddened by the crying I heard on the other end when I picked up. But this time, there were no fevers involved, no blood, and no diarrhea in her explanation.

"Kelly Ripa and Michael Strahan are going to read my name on TV tomorrow! I was selected as a finalist in their Teacher of the Year search! Besides you, my former students and their parents also wrote letters on my behalf. Can you believe it? This is incredible!"

I could feel her thankfulness, astonishment, and humility through the phone while she explained what was going to happen. It was not lost on us that she had almost died not once but twice and now the sun was truly shining on her, and for damn good reasons. She's a hell of a teacher. In fact, she's been teaching me things my whole life: how to rollerblade, how to sneak out *and* get caught, how to keep a desirable closet, how to be thoughtful, how to have fun, how to be a good parent, and how to roll with life's punches. And most importantly, how to recover from being dealt an unlucky hand with a gracious and enviable attitude.

Time stopped for all of us when we tuned into the show the following morning. They waited until the last minutes to discuss the contest and Danielle's name was one of the first to be read by Kelly.

"From Salamanca, New York, Mrs. Danielle Eaton!"

When her face was put up on the screen I screamed with glee! To see our girl on live TV with the entire country watching gave me such a sense of pride and joy. At her school, they stopped classes and allowed everyone to watch it in their rooms. Even in May's pre-kindergarten class, the teacher stopped to tune in live. I'm positive I got little or no work done the rest of the day as I lobbied everyone I knew, and then everyone they knew, to get online and vote for her. Despite my burgeoning belly, I was bound and determined to go to New York City and see her win, and it looked like she was in the running to become one of the two finalists based on the votes we saw. Though we probably didn't eat much because we were too excited, we all gathered that evening at a local diner when everyone got home from work. We planned with delight and reviewed the prior day's events. In reliving these moments, there seemed to be an electricity in the air. Everything was happening so fast. The energy was positive but intense.

What we did not account for in our furious push to get people to vote was that the number of comments under each candidate mattered to the competition. Although she had one of the highest number of votes cast, she did not win in the comments column. Thus, the next morning when we all tuned in again to see who it was narrowed down to, we were disappointed Danielle Eaton was left out of the mix. Throughout the hectic 48 hours that had ensued, Danielle was calm, proud, and never got ahead of herself, akin to a nice, warm slice of humble pie. She contended that she was grateful to be included and with total certainty, I know she genuinely meant that. She knew what it was like to almost lose it all and so this was just a cherry on the hot fudge sundae (she really likes hot fudge sundaes) she already considered her life to be. I, on the other hand, was extremely sad that she had come so close and didn't reap the full recognition that I thought she deserved. But, as the years passed, I came to agree with her. So what if she didn't make it to New York City? Our community, her school, and most notably, our family, knew who she was and what she accomplished as an educator – the most vital part of that job – to positively impact the kids who look to their teacher for guidance and validation that they matter. Danielle had certainly won that prize without the help of Kelly Ripa and Michael Strahan.

CHAPTER 5

Her rise to fame came to a halt just as quickly as it started. The ride was fun, though, and I can now say it was worth every minute. It was an exciting shock to our small-town systems and the type of adrenaline that we'd much rather have over an unexpected trip to the hospital. I went on to have my son, Sawyer, in early June and time marched on for all of us. The days and months moved us forward into 2016 and towards the sparkle a new year brings.

Danielle had been on Asacol since 2012 with no issues – no blood, no diarrhea, no painful abdomen. Nothing. Nada. Zilch. She was in full remission!

Until her insurance company decided to spice things up.

If you are so inclined to raise your blood pressure, Google "why are drugs dropped from insurance companies?" and you will discover some frightening statistics. The percentage that this occurs seems to be increasing greatly, much to the detriment of patients. I would hope that there is a fantastic reason that doesn't include padded bank accounts but after my quick search, I am not a believer that there is any altruism at play.

Thus, Danielle received a letter before Christmas in 2015 that Asacol would no longer be available to her and that she needed to find an alternative option. Just what she was hoping Santa would leave for her under the tree, a major medicine switch four years into remission. She didn't fret, though, and simply contacted her GI doctor for a plan of action. They settled on a non-sulfa drug, Lialda, that would hopefully fill the strong shoes Asacol had left behind. Her doctor told her that it was identical to Asacol and it would be covered by her insurance.

She filled the prescription and made it through January, all of February, *and* through BillFest2016, with no issues whatsoever.

You're familiar with BillFest2016, right?

Well, in case you live under a rock, it's like Coachella...if Coachella were in a rural Upstate New York town and didn't involve celebrities of any kind or fancy concerts.

However, it was still a rockin' good time. BillFest2016 was the careful result of months and months of planning. A fête to be remembered for generations. Bill happened to be born on February 29th (Leap Year) in 1976 thus he was turning the big 4-0 in 2016. And because she does nothing sub-par, BillFest was a magnificent night of surprises planned solely by Danielle, for the merriment of her husband. She had rented a party bus and had Bill's family and friends from all over the country secretly fly into town. They were strategically placed along the party bus' route of bars and taverns. In a nutshell, there were specially made koozies, five bar stops, a Black Eyed Peas dance off at 2:00 in the morning, and a vomiting party-goer; all the makings of an unforgettable evening. It went off without a hitch.

Sunday rolled around, though, and she saw it, just

24 hours after her monumental surprise party for Bill, one single drop of blood made itself known in her toilet. It was not accompanied by any other uncomfortable symptoms but it was there nonetheless. She did not panic and had learned her lesson (thank God!) not to sit on it. Her two prior hospital stays taught her that she could not toughen up and ride it out. She made an appointment the following week to discuss what she had seen with her GI doctor.

His first line of defense was to have her take steroids, in a pill form, to see if that would lessen the inflammation. Their joint hope was that it was a small setback and the magic of Prednisone would shrink her colon back to normal. Yet, as each day passed, the lone drop of blood brought a friend and they eventually brought even more friends to the fantastic toilet party occurring in her bathroom each time she had to go.

February ran into March like a slow downhill train, moving along at turtle speed. Gradual but still very powerful and picking up momentum along the way. It caused things to sour for her once more. She didn't want to admit it but her body was beginning to turn on her like it had in the past.

Her new routine of bloody bathroom occurrences had her continually keeping up with her doctor on a regular basis. Because her symptoms were progressing in the wrong direction, he decided that he needed a better picture of what was going on so he scheduled her for a colonoscopy. Colonoscopies had become a normal part of Danielle's annual wellness routine even when she was in remission because, unfortunately, those with UC are at a greater risk of developing colon cancer down the road.

Scheduling a colonoscopy during a flare up, though, is always a risk for the patient. By inserting a scope into a diseased colon, there is a danger of moving that infection around and allowing it to take a detour via your bloodstream. Essentially, that is what happened to her in the first go-around. Sepsis had set in because the disease moved past her colon and into her blood. It was clear that the steroids were not strong enough and they needed to be certain how severe the situation was.

The test confirmed what they knew, this was a true flare up and some ulcers were present.

Because she was already taking a medicine to help suppress her wonky immune response, in addition to the steroids, but was clearly having a relapse, her doctor prescribed another medication. The add-on was a booster of sorts to help the UC medicine really do its job. The goal for the new medicine was to give her system a stronger push to calm the heck down and allow the flare up to recede. She filled the prescription and hoped that it would do its job.

April appeared, though, and so did the bloody stool that was still fully cemented in her daily routine. Midway through the month we celebrated my birthday with our entire family over Chinese food and gourmet cupcakes. After the last egg roll had been eaten, Danielle, our mother and I, went outside in the inviting April sun and chatted about Danielle's rear end.

"Danielle, how are you feeling? Are you beginning to get nervous?" I asked. I knew the answers to both questions but it felt like she was teetering on the edge of tears and maybe she wanted to release some of her worries.

"I am," she said.

Yet she spoke about having a plan and looking to her GI doctor for answers. She hoped with this plan in place that she would not end up wearing a hospital gown and eating mushy meatloaf on a cafeteria tray anytime soon. My mom and I pumped her full of positive affirmations but had our fingers crossed behind our backs. We had no idea what we were up against and no real assurance that she was headed for recovery and remission.

I remember having a lovely time at that birthday gathering and being grateful for my life. But I also remember feeling crestfallen. The realization that she was sick and scared had settled in because she openly admitted it to the universe. It was out there in the ether and that meant it had weight.

Spring break came shortly thereafter and Danielle had big plans for her time off that revolved around her work. Unfortunately, her school's future was hanging in the balance of a state analysis. As a district, their graduation rates were down and their test scores were low, which meant that there was a real possibility the school could be shut down and run by the state. In order to fully assess the situation, the state was going to be visiting her school and would be observing every single teacher and classroom. To help do her part, Danielle had great intentions of creating the best lessons she could on the Holocaust and JFK for the two classes for which she would be observed. She had bought a swanky new outfit, a new pair of shoes, and was looking forward to working every morning of her break to make both lessons engaging and educational. She's a morning person and loves the first sips of her coffee, the feel of comfortable pajamas, and the clicking of her keyboard when her thoughts are the most focused. Yet, when she sat down on her first day off, she took her sip and was immediately driven to the bathroom. Her UC also subscribed to the notion that the early bird gets the worm. Oftentimes it was in full swing in those early morning hours. What could have been a relaxing and productive week of work took Danielle twice as long and was incredibly frustrating and painful. After each trip to the commode, the pain clock would start and for about 45 minutes after going, she would experience the internal discomfort that occurs when you release poop through a bloody and raw area.

Her large bowel had started to shred itself.

She was disheartened with her relapse but more so because her annual mid-May trip to Washington D.C. with 40 eighth graders was also looming and she knew the complications UC would create. She launched the Washington D.C. Club when she started teaching at Salamanca and had been the group's fearless leader ever since. She had wonderful support from other teachers and school staff but Danielle was the Chief-in-Charge. As the month wore on and her symptoms worsened, she finally broke down and began to panic. How could she let these students down and the parents who looked to her to keep their kids safe while away from home in a major metropolitan city?

As she tried to make sense of what she was going to do with the trip, she simultaneously made the realization that something else might be going on with her bowel. The frequency that she was going increased tenfold in a very short amount of time. She had come to understand what UC felt like but this seemed like a distant cousin to UC. Her doctor was also keenly paying attention to her symptoms. He decided to test her for C. *diff* to see if that was the culprit for the radically increased amount of bathroom trips she was now taking.

C. *diff* is a bacterium that also causes diarrhea and inflammation of the colon and often results when the normal bacterial flora of the bowel change. How fantastic for her, because she tested positive for it! It is an interesting bug because it can live in your colon for a long time, just relaxing in there, without presenting any of its awful symptoms. You can pick it up just about anywhere and, in fact, hospitals are a common place to catch it. And if you happen to take an antibiotic for another ailment, it can kill all of the good bacteria also hanging out down there which allows the C. *diff* monsters to rise up and wreak havoc.

To add in some perspective, she was still teaching from 7:00 in the morning to 3:00 in the afternoon every day. A long day at the outset but realistically, her schedule looked like this: the alarm rang at the glorious time of 4:47 so she could get herself ready, correct papers, have coffee, and be out the door by 6:40 to make it to school by 7:00. Then she taught on her feet all day and usually got home between 3:30 and 4:00 when she then had to put her "mom" hat back on and tend to Lily and May, who were eight and six. She had to help with homework, make dinner, tie up any loose ends she had for work the following day, and then try to crawl into bed at a decent hour.

Earlier in the book, I asked you to imagine her circumstances as if they were yours and once again, I'd like you play along. Picture yourself trotting through that same day, but having to stop abruptly and run to the bathroom anywhere from eight to 15 times a day. Fifteen times, people! That is not an exaggeration because almost every morning my mom and I would text her or call for the tally and daily update to see how bad it had gotten. Usually, things were worse in the evening and at night, when her body would slow down, which meant that she did not always (actually almost rarely during that time) get a reprieve once she fell asleep. Her body would wake her up and force her to the bathroom, sometimes two or three times in a night. Pure exhaustion was starting to become her normal state of being and a dark, gray cloud slowly crept in, yet again, over her life.

I started to have an inkling of how rotten things were for her based on our regular morning text messages to one another. I am a notoriously poor sleeper. It's one of my super powers. Four hours of sleep for me is not ideal but it's also not a major problem. For Danielle, and most people above the age of 25, it would cause quite the obstruction to having a pleasant day. Here is a sampling of what those messages entailed over the course of a week in early May of 2016:

Me: Morning, how did you sleep last night?

Danielle: Not horrible! I had to get up a couple of times but then went right back to bed. Smiley face emoji.

Red flag number one - having to get up in the middle of the night to empty your colon. That is not a common activity nor is it normal nocturnal behavior.

Me: Buongiorno! Was last night any better for you? Fingers crossed emoji.

Danielle: Last night was ok. I was up four times and needed to take some pain medicine because my rear end is sore. I'll lie down after school though! Wink face emoji.

Red flag number two - we are not a family who naps. For right or for wrong, napping was for sissies or if you were sick. And my sister was not a sissy.

Me: Top of the mornin' to ya. Please tell me you slept better last night?

Danielle: It wasn't terrible. No emoji.

Red flag number three - no emoji. She was and is a very upbeat text messenger. You can hear the positivity emanate through her words. But, by this point in the game, she had the texting intonation of Eeyore on his worst day.

Because her sleep was becoming so disrupted, she had to admit a slight amount of defeat and go to her vice principal. With very few details given on her end, she let him know she wasn't entirely healthy and might need to leave early on occasion to make her doctor's appointments. He was very sympathetic to her plight as a Crohn's soldier himself. She was relieved to have his support and the peace of mind that she could leave to get to doctor's appointments since it's hard to snag the coveted after 3:00 spots that teachers need.

She was not relieved, though, as she thought about her D.C. trip which was just days away. In the back of her mind, she knew she wasn't healthy enough to go but she was still holding onto hope that once the C. diff worked its way out, she would turn the corner and start to feel better. She had to wave the white flag once more and admit to her principal, in addition to the vice principal, that she had an untimely affliction causing some disruption in her life.

"I just wanted to let you know that I have this disease called ulcerative colitis. As bad luck would have it, it has decided to make a comeback. I will be fine to go on the trip, but I just wanted you to be aware of what was going on and that I may need to take a day or two off once I get back."

An awkward pause ensued.

Then he asked, "are you sure you should go?"

She assured him that she was still capable of making the trek to our nation's capital despite what she was fighting internally. Overall, he was supportive and Danielle felt better looping him in, even if it meant having to disclose a very personal issue.

My mother and I were back to biting our nails and nervously smoking imaginary cigarettes each night in total terror of this trip. It was extremely obvious to the naked eye that she was unwell and the thought of her on a seven-hour bus ride with adolescents seemed to silently scream "danger" in our opinion. Not to mention the two more strenuous days of non-stop walking that would follow. She's a tough, part-Polish, part-Sicilian gal, though, and willed herself the ability to take this trip. She made the decision she was going to go, but with the caveat that she could get her own hotel room. She rationalized that if she was able to get a single room instead of sharing with another chaperone, she would have the private bathroom she needed and the ability to rest better during the very little rest time that the trip afforded. We relented, prayed for the best, and off she went.

Their sojourn south through Pennsylvania and

Virginia started for Danielle at 4:00 in the morning. She made it to the school by 5:00 and the bus left at 6:00. She powered through the long ride and was feeling okay but ready for some alone time on the commode. The first hurdle appeared, though, when they went to check into their hotel. The hotel's front desk clerk shared the following very ill-fated news with Danielle who was anxiously awaiting her private bathroom.

"I'm sorry, Mrs. Eaton, we do not have a single room for you at this time."

"What? I called last week and reserved my own room and received confirmation that it had been secured."

Instead of bursting into tears like she wanted to do, Danielle asked her tour guide for help. In prior years she had been paired with repeat guides, but on this trip, she was given a new one. While the kids milled about and found their rooms, Danielle once again had to share the news of her colon conundrum with the guide.

Without missing a beat, the guide was sympathetic and empathetic.

"I only have half of my colon! I completely understand."

It turns out that the guide, a lovely woman in her early fifties, had faced colon cancer when she was younger and was fully aware of the mayhem colon troubles can cause for a person.

They then worked together with the front desk to correct the unfortunate error. It took about 30 minutes of finagling but Danielle and her new BFF tour guide were able to find her a private room. However, all of the back and forth ate into the small, precious bit of personal time Danielle required. The show needed to go on, though, and the 8th graders were ready to bust a move. They all piled back into buses and headed to the Potomac River for a dinner and dancing cruise. I was a chaperone on this trip in 2018, and let me tell you, folks, the kids loved that dinner cruise.

The same rang true in 2016. Her students were having the time of their lives away from home. They danced, sang, and let their inhibitions go. Danielle was happy to have been there to see it and to know that so much hard work throughout the year had paid off. She held onto that feeling over the next 48 hours, as things did not go as smoothly as planned.

For starters, four students succumbed to a stomach bug and were forced to call their parents and be picked up early from D.C. It was the first time that had ever happened and everyone involved was extremely disappointed that the trip was cut short for the kids. The first kid went down before the cruise ship disembarked from the harbor. Alexis, who was a chaperone on the trip, offered to stay back with him.

On the morning of day two, the second kid came down with it. He threw up but tried to rally as they headed to the Capitol building. Danielle warned him that they wouldn't be able to get back to the bus for another six hours, so if he felt nauseous, he needed to make the decision right then to leave or be forced to stick with the group for the majority of the day. He didn't want to miss out despite being three shades of green. He threw up again with no container to catch it. Danielle then pleaded with the groundskeepers at the Capitol for a trash bag.

She described the scenario as a funny one all these years later, as the poor student had to carry around an industrial-sized black garbage bag (i.e., a landscaping bag) for the rest of the tour just in case the gag reflex appeared again.

Danielle tried to make the best of the day as well, but things went sideways for her. The itinerary had them visiting the very large and beautiful Pentagon City Mall followed by a fantastic play, "Shear Madness," at the Kennedy Center. In healthy times, Danielle utilized every single second of the shopping time to browse, try on, and purchase items to add to her closet. As I mentioned earlier, she's a purveyor of fine garments and treats herself whenever she has the opportunity. On this trip, however, she treated herself to the swanky bathroom in Nordstrom's for the duration of their time there. Once her system decided it was time to "go" she was a slave to the toilet. And if that wasn't awful enough, her pain began to increase with each evacuation. It became apparent to her that things were not improving and in fact were getting worse. She called Bill and confided in him.

"Bill, I'm in trouble."

He sensed the dread in her voice, and like the supportive husband that he is, he assured her they would get through it and would tackle her troubles as soon as she got home. She collected herself and her stuff, put a smile on her face, and headed to the designated meeting spot where she learned that another poor student had gotten the stomach flu.

To the third kid who got sick at the mall that night, I'm so sorry. But really, I'd like to thank you and buy you a cookie. Because you were stricken ill, it "forced" Danielle to take one for the team and escort you back to the hotel where she was then able to skip the play and rest all night long.

When Friday morning dawned on day number three, kid number four went down for the count. The chaperones had set up a sick room the night before and quarantined the other three together until their parents could come and pick them up. Unfortunately for kid number four, he was sent home that day, too.

Another "unfortunately" is in order. One would think that having to muster the energy to be the leader of this group would be tough enough, but we know Danielle was also fighting the silent UC battle as well. And to add insult to injury on day number three, she had to contend with an angry chaperone from another school who did not take the time to understand the situation fully before placing judgment.

As she was walking one of the sick kids to the car to be driven home, with her arm around his shoulder for comfort, she was approached and accosted by a man who had clearly eaten rocks for breakfast. He glanced down at her t-shirt, which stated the name of her school, and then began a bitter diatribe at the lack of respect her students had for others.

"Can you not control your students? We heard doors closing at all hours of the night and students shuffling back and forth. That is totally unacceptable!"

Danielle's deep-rooted frustration for all things occurring in that moment (the unlucky, sick kids going home and missing out on the last day, her misfortune for being born with a defective colon, and the asshole now standing before her) rushed to the surface of her consciousness. But instead of letting him have it, she carefully and concisely communicated her mood by snarling two simple words.

"BACK. OFF."

As a good Italian woman, she would have liked to use profanity in place of "back," but her good, Italian teacher mind prevailed.

Captain Jerk Chaperone did not back down, however, and did not retreat from the situation at that moment, like he should have. What he didn't know, though, is that Alexis and Danielle, like all best friends, vibrate on the same frequency and have a sixth sense when trouble is in the water. Alexis looked up from what she was doing and immediately came flying to Danielle's aid. She knew that this man was clearly out of line and barking up the wrong tree. Without asking any questions she conjured up the very best gesture to meet that moment. She stuck her hand in front of his face and in a very childish, but perfect motion, kept closing it repeatedly as if to verbally say to him, "Shut your God forsaken lips!"

Finally, after Alexis' interruption, he realized that he was going to be defeated in his quest to ruin their day.

Had he asked respectfully what could have occurred the night before, they would have explained to him that there were sick children and they needed to move them around so they could be put together. They would have also told Captain Jerk that they hired security to patrol the halls all night long and that when the sick kid came out of his room, the security guard was all over it and they went to get Alexis together.

After the rude occurrence, the student who had been with Danielle looked up at her with kind and grateful eyes.

"Thank you, Mrs. Eaton. I can't believe that just happened."

"I can't either," she said with a smirk.

The sordid tale did not end there. After the sick kids were sent off, the rest of the group boarded their buses and headed off to Arlington National Cemetery. It is a beautifully peaceful space that requires no cell phones to be in use while you are visiting, especially when you are witnessing the tranquil wreath laying ritual at the tomb of the Unknown Soldier. Danielle is normally very good about switching off her phone, but in the commotion of the morning she had forgotten and her phone began to ring.

And it wasn't Avon calling.

It was her principal.

"Danielle, is there a discipline problem that I need to know about?"

"Discipline problem? No. I have no idea what you are talking about?"

"I just got off the phone with a chaperone from another school who said that our kids were being disrespectful and were up at all hours of the night."

"Oh geez."

Captain Jerk had noticed her shirt, googled the number, and called the principal.

"No, there wasn't a problem at all," she explained.

"It was the sick kids we had to send home. We decided to quarantine them together so we switched some around in the middle of the night. The security guards alerted us and everything was taken care of within an hour."

He, of course, believed her and she could prove it because the security company requires each guard to do a lap up and down the hallway every 15 minutes and log their findings, or lack thereof.

She was grateful that her principal had her back and that she wasn't getting detention for being a bad group leader, but she had to circle back to her silent opponent, UC. Despite the sick kids and the hiccup she had already dealt with, it was clear to Danielle that after Arlington she would not get to spend her day perusing a Smithsonian Museum, the next item on the agenda. Instead, she had the great privilege of checking out the fine art on the back of bathroom stalls.

Right off the bat, upon arriving there, she had the urge to go and needed to do something quick. Yet, she was waiting in line for her group to get through security. She was filled with fear at the idea of not getting to a bathroom quick enough. Before she could formulate a plan, the universe did her a solid and her BFF tour guide helped her once again when she noticed the discomfort written on Danielle's face.

"Danielle, are you needing to use the restroom?"

"Yes ma'am, I really do."

"If you leave your backpack with me, I'll wait and go through security with all of the kids and you can jump ahead to the line for people without bags and go right through. You'll get in much quicker that way."

"Oh my goodness! Thank you so much!"

Danielle scurried ahead and made it in the nick of time. She spent almost the entire day bouncing from bathroom to bathroom while the kids toured the various museum mainstays of D.C. After lunch, while sitting on a bench waiting for the students to huddle up before departing for home, Alexis and Danielle found themselves sharing in a quiet moment between best friends. Until this point, Alexis had respected the unspoken rule between the two of them on the trip: do not discuss the "colon" in the room, that Danielle was in serious trouble. Danielle put her wearied head on Alexis' shoulder and Alexis put her arm around Danielle to let her know that she saw what she was silently going through.

"It's going to be okay, buddy. It's going to be okay."

As in other times throughout Danielle's journey when someone would utter those same words, neither Alexis nor Danielle was really sure if that was true or not. But on that D.C. bench, they both needed to believe it and have hope that there was some truth to what Alexis said and that she would eventually be okay.

By the time the bus arrived to drive them back home, Danielle's bottom was sore, she was physically exhausted, and was ready to take a seat. Despite her noisy eighth grade companions, she was able to rest. She remembered, though, that when the bus got back to the school around midnight the school wouldn't be open like she had planned. Because she's a mom, a teacher, and someone with an uncontrollable rectum, prior to departing, she had asked a parent, who is also the elementary school's assistant principal, if when they came to pick up their son on Friday evening, they could open up the school so "people" could use the bathroom before going home. It just so happened this was one of the parents who had to come and get their son earlier that day because of the stomach flu, so they weren't going to be there to unlock it.

Best laid plans.

She gritted her teeth, talked herself into being okay for the 25 or so minutes that she had to wait on the drive from the school to her house and set off for home. She pulled into the driveway, sprinted to the front door, and did not make it. After an already depleting day, she now had to contend with an accident at almost 1:00 in the morning. The dark cloud over her had gotten a little darker.

Her eyes opened the next morning to the chirping sounds of Lily and May. Danielle was extremely grateful to be home and even thought to herself, "I don't feel that bad right now." She started her day by making a cup of coffee, talking to our Gram who called to see how she was feeling, and told the girls she'd give them their presents over breakfast. The girls were tickled to have their mom home because that meant she had neat gifts for them acquired during her trip. Halfway through her toast, though, there it was, her canary in the coal mine, the urge to go to the bathroom.

As the early morning turned into the afternoon, she continued to feel worse and had already gone to the bathroom 6-10 times.

She knew what she needed to do. The ulcerative

colitis was winning the battle and she needed to surrender and wave her trusty white flag once more. First, she lay in bed hoping against hope that this was a nightmare she'd wake up from. When that miracle didn't happen, she placed a call she did not want to make but knew it was the right thing to do.

"Mom, I'm really not feeling well."

In Danielle's fairy tale universe, she suggested that she might just need to eat some lunch and take a nap, and if she was still not better, maybe they could go to the ER.

My mother, however, did not have wings and certainly did not live in fairy-tale-land. She responded as such.

"Bullshit. I'm coming over right now."

My mom hopped into her car and headed towards Danielle's home. It's only 10 minutes away but as she neared her house, the rainstorm that had been brewing all morning finally released its fury. The rain became blinding, the wind whipped, and the thunder was startling. My impatient mother wanted to drive 95 mph down the semi-rural road but because of the torrential precipitation, she was forced to go very slow. In retrospect, the storm was a theatrical addition to the gravity of the situation. It's as if those gray clouds that had been hovering over Danielle for months finally hit their breaking point as well.

She arrived a few minutes later, took one look at her oldest daughter, and said:

"We're calling the doctor right now. I'm not messing around with a nap and some lunch."

My mom describes Danielle's state as "terrifying." When she walked into Danielle's bedroom, Danielle was lying in the fetal position. Her face had no color and she looked severely ill. Even though it was Saturday, they were able to reach Danielle's favorite PCP doctor, who instructed them to head directly to the emergency room.

For obvious reasons, Bill was on kid duty and had to shuttle them to a birthday party before he could drop them off at his mom's and meet my mother at the ER. Danielle's pain level was almost intolerable, but upon arriving at the hospital, they were able to give her pain meds to squelch its intensity. A peace washed over her like a warm bath and she was finally able to submit to the situation and let the nurses and doctors take over.

Thankfully, she wasn't in the ER too long before they admitted her and brought her up to a room on the 3rd floor of the hospital, the surgical floor. Danielle was going to need another colonoscopy and they needed to prep for it. But this third-floor room was not a private room. Luckily, a kind soul moved some things around shortly after her admission and was able to get her a private room on the 2nd floor. Although she was headed for a colonoscopy, she was also someone that had just tested positive for C. diff, and the hospital preferred to keep a patient like that confined to her own room. Hooray for the small victories of not having to share a hospital room (and subsequently a commode).

By this time, doctors knew what they were up against. But they needed to understand the significance of this flare up, so a colonoscopy, despite its risks, was the next step. After a couple of days there, she was rested enough to start the preparation for it. As I mentioned earlier, for a healthy person getting ready for a colonoscopy, a beverage laden with a laxative aid must be consumed in order to completely empty your bowels, which allows the doctors to get a good look at the environment inside your intestinal walls. In this case, though, Danielle was not well enough to tolerate that method so they had to revert back to her old pal, the warm water enema.

My mom, bless her nurse heart, knew that she could assist Danielle and walk her through having to perform an enema on herself, but, in her mind, she was desperately wishing Steve were there by her side. She wanted his unending moral support as a husband and his physician's knowledge for guidance.

He was, however, on the other side of the world in Cambodia with Madison who had studied abroad in Singapore for the Spring semester of 2016. And as bad luck would have it, just before Danielle left for D.C., Steve flew to Singapore to pick up Madison and tour Southeast Asia with her. It wasn't feasible for them to cut their trip short and fly home early so, unfortunately, Steve had to do his best to be there for my mom albeit a 12-hour time difference separating them.

So, there my mom stood, on the other side of the bathroom door, telling Danielle what do with each step of the uncomfortable process. Armed with three bags of warm tap water (each being about one liter) Danielle had the very unpleasant job of inserting a tube inside her own rectum to allow the water to flow in. Danielle cried in agony while my mom silently whimpered to herself on the other side of the door.

"Danielle, just think of the spring flowers we can buy when you get out of here. We'll go as soon as you're home and pick up beautiful perennials. Pinks, whites, purples. Geraniums, begonias. And why don't we plan a nice dinner once you're back on your feet? We'll all go and celebrate."

My mom desperately tried to deflect and change the subject to anything other than what they were currently doing. It was a hard feat to overcome, though. With each release of water into her rear end, the pain was merciless. Danielle tried to hold it in as long as she could but her poor body ultimately gave up. All that came out was blood and water.

The results of the scope reflected what Danielle had been feeling and what anyone who looked at her could sense, that she was in the throes of a major UC relapse and she needed a new plan.

Pause here for a moment and go check out the alarming colonoscopy images from May of 2016.

Awful, right?

At this point in the story, her GI doctor suggested that it might be prudent to try another classification of drugs called biologics because she needed another solution. Although she technically could have gone back to her tried and true workhorse of a medicine, Asacol, it still wasn't covered and they would once again be out of pocket $702 a month. Plus, the doctor believed that the Lialda was incredibly similar to Asacol and it had failed her. The only other type of pill medication that was available to her were the sulfas and those were obviously off the table.

If you're not familiar with biologics, you have probably seen the commercials for them, which include:

Humira, Entyvio, and Remicade. Biologics are medications that are created from a biological source, something that was or is living. They have been proven to work with reducing inflammation and targeting specific tissues versus serving the whole body. They are usually administered via an infusion and are the next line of defense against UC when oral medications stop being effective.

Like most things, there are two sides to the story with regard to this type of medication. Some people in our inner circle had serious reservations about the end result if Danielle were to get the infusions. At the time, I was oblivious to the potentially unpleasant side effects that could occur. If I was aware of them, I might have just filed away the list of possible side effects as something the drug companies just have to list in case they are sued.

Now, after some time and research, I know that at a minimum, biologics do diminish the healthy parts of a patient's immune system, which can cause a host of horrendous problems to occur. In other words, the goal of these medications is to dampen down one's own immune system so it stops fighting itself. Think of it this way, before you begin taking them, you start with an immune system army of 100,000 combat soldiers who are beating up your colon for no good reason. In order to curb the damage they are causing, you re-assign 50,000 of those lieutenants to R & R for the weekend. But by doing that, you become more susceptible to getting sick because your battalion isn't as robust any longer. It's the classic challenge of, "which is the lesser of two evils?" Do you expose yourself to the possibility of being sick with other pathogens or do you allow your immune system to keep up its assault?

The most common ailments that afflict those who are administered biologics are colds and respiratory infections, with tuberculosis also on the list of possibilities. I wanted to add this information as a quasi-PSA. Folks, just do your homework and look into the prescription you were given and how it could affect whichever autoimmune disorder with which you were blessed.

Danielle opted to move forward with the biologic infusions because she was running out of options. It can take a while for paperwork to be filed, the insurance company to approve, and the infusion appointment to be set. But, by the grace of the UC gods, Danielle was able to receive her first infusion shortly after she was released from hospital stay number three. My mom took her to the first appointment, where she sat in a chair for four hours, attached to an IV.

Then we waited. And prayed. And waited. And prayed some more.

We were desperate for this medication to work and to be the panacea for her ailment. She did not improve noticeably before she received the second infusion. Her bottom was still pretty sore and she was still not at her best. So, when our father took her to the second appointment a week later, she got more than she bargained for on the ride there. Because he was a former beer distributor who hauled beer trailers full of kegs, at that time he drove an enormous diesel pickup truck. And when that behemoth took a bump, poor Danielle felt it. By the time she reached the doctor's office, she was in agony. We then waited yet again after the second infusion for her to turn a corner and start to feel better.

When Danielle, despite her soreness and weak demeanor, discussed going back to work so she could end the school year with her students, my mom and I broke out our imaginary Marlboros because we both felt it was too soon and she was pushing it. Why risk getting sick again to go back to work at the very end of the school year? We underestimated Danielle's commitment to her students, though, and her drive to be a good employee. Kelly Ripa and Michael Strahan had said her name on national TV, damnit. She was hell-bent on being normal and not missing out on any more weeks of her life. So, by mid-June, and only a month post-hospital stay, she tried to go back to work.

Did she make it to the end of the school year with her students?

Nope.

She didn't even make it a full week. The pain was still there. She was still going to the bathroom a ton and wasn't sleeping through the night, too many variables to juggle in order to make it through an eight-hour workday teaching the aspiring minds of tomorrow.

But she was bound and determined to make it to her 20th high school reunion, which fell on the Friday of the same week she tried to go back to teaching. She dug down deep inside and donned a beautiful pink sun dress with gold accents. She applied snazzy going-out make up and curled her hair. I happened to have also been in attendance at the alumni dinner that night, because it was my 15-year class reunion. Sitting across from her, you would not have been able to guess she was secretly sick inside. She looked gorgeous and the closest to her normal self that I had seen in a long time. If you look at pictures from that evening, though, it's evident that she was on the thin side due to her very visible protruding collarbone. She carefully ate the meal she was served, hoping not to eat something that would cause her innards to revolt against her. But as soon as the meal concluded, she wilted and needed to get home immediately for fear of an accident. She missed out on the fun that was to happen afterwards. As she begged off, one of her friends commented on how wonderful (and thin) she looked. "Oh girlfriend, if only your compliment was true for the right reasons," she thought sadly to herself.

Bill drove the few miles home while Danielle tried to clench her rear end tightly. She ran to the door and once again, did not make it inside before her body unleashed its fury all over her and that beautiful pink sun dress with gold accents.

During this stretch of time, Danielle's only medication to combat the pain is something called Tramadol. In the world of narcotic painkillers, it is fairly weak. For someone who has to live in immense pain around the clock, it is not always efficacious. Danielle jokingly referred to them as Sweet Tarts after she was introduced to someone else whose autoimmune disorder, Rheumatoid Arthritis (RA), kept them in constant agony as well. When Danielle told the acquaintance that she was getting by on Tramadol alone, his response gave her a good laugh.

"Tramadol too? It's like taking a Sweet Tart, right? Not very effective at all."

Both she and the RA sufferer knew that consistent, heavy narcotic use was a dangerous path but the weaker alternative, Tramadol, didn't cut it. Taking painkillers on a regular basis is not something that she took lightly in any way. As a family, we have personally been touched by the fatal consequences of opioid misuse and the disease of addiction, the effects of which are tragic and eternal. Sadly, we lost our first cousin, who was in his mid-twenties and had just become a father, to the opioid epidemic and Danielle never forgot that. But in a world that felt void of happiness, playfully using the name "Sweet Tart" allowed her to crack a smile every now and again.

While Tramadol wasn't too potent, she was careful to never drive while taking it. Compared to heavy hitters like Morphine or Dilaudid, Tramadol was the tame sibling. This is worth noting because this short section of her story could be categorized as "Chapter Pain." Every day she suffered an agonizing pain sensation that rarely abated. She was in constant contact with her GI doctor's office and was told, "If you are in intense, unending pain, you either need to be seen ASAP or admitted to the hospital."

She grinned (not really, because what was there to grin about?) and took it because being re-admitted seemed worse than dealing with the pain in the comforts of her own home. During Chapter Pain, her doctor also happened to be out of the country because his father, who lived overseas, had become ill. But because he knew how sick she was, he checked in with his office regularly, something he deserves a chocolate chip cookie for, as well.

Also, during Chapter Pain, our brother Noah (the progeny of my mom and step-dad, Steve) graduated high school. My first memory of that day was standing on the school's steps waiting for Danielle and Bill to arrive so I could give them their tickets. It was a delightful, sunny June morning and as soon as I saw Danielle approaching, it suddenly felt bleak. She did not have joy written anywhere on her face and my heart began to sink. She had a dress on, but appeared as if she'd rather have been at home in bed under a blanket. In recalling that day, she admits the smiles she shared were forced. She was in too much pain to sit and watch from her seat, so she stood in the back of the auditorium the whole time.

When the ceremony ended, there was a break in time before we headed to our favorite restaurant 30 minutes away, Villagio. She used that time to go home and lay down until the absolute last second before they had to meet us. Driving to the restaurant she wished and hoped that she could feel normal and enjoy a nice meal with a little vino and some lively conversations with family.

Heck, she wanted to order things with seeds! To get a little wild and crazy and eat something spicy or, better yet, greasy. It would have been a dream. She played it safe mostly but did imbibe some wine so that she could experience something semi-normal. Dinner went okay until the kids wanted to get ice cream across the street. She had to rush back to the restaurant and use the bathroom and basically never rejoined our group again. She went home and had one of the worst nights she had ever incurred up until that point.

She paced in their living room all night long. Back and forth she walked, gritting her teeth and clenching her fists to try and get past the throbbing pain taking over her body. Sometimes a hot bath squelched the pain temporarily. So, even though it was a warm summer night, she periodically would get in and out of the tub. By morning, she was completely worn-out. My mom called to check in and see how the night had been for her since she knew it hadn't ended well at the restaurant.

"Good morning, how did you do last night?" she asked.

A pregnant pause ensued.

There weren't many occasions where Danielle broke down and shared really what she was thinking and feeling but this morning was one of those times. Her stiff upper lip softened as the tears fell.

She sobbed into the phone.

"Mom, I am in so much pain. It's more than I can handle. I was up all night without any real relief. I paced and cried like an animal stuck in a cage."

Bill would later reflect on these nights by admitting that he knew it was a bad night for her when she would have to go out to the living room to try to sleep. When he woke up and saw the heating pad and the blankets strewn about the couch, sadness would set in. He was a powerless husband watching his wife deteriorate, mentally and physically, right before his eyes.

CHAPTER 6

Let's walk down memory lane for a minute and share Bill and Danielle's love story. One can only take so much depressing colon content without a break!

He was a good Catholic boy who went to the only private Catholic high school in town, Archbishop Walsh, while Danielle went to the public school, Olean High. Though the schools were separate during the week, the students intermingled when Friday and Saturday nights rolled around. However, in our small town, teenage entertainment was minimal. For example, cow tipping is an actual option because there isn't much to do. Therefore, generations of high school kids have gathered together on weekends to drink cheap beer out of a Solo cup and let their inhibitions go. One magical Friday night when Danielle was 15 and Bill was 17, after meeting at a house party, she set her sights on ensnaring him.

It was 1994, Beck's "Loser" was playing in the background and Danielle remembers spotting him from across the room. Bill was sporting a J. Crew-esque look that included a polo shirt, sandy brown hair parted to the side, glasses, and a genuine smile. They exchanged pleasantries and Danielle was able to snag his telephone number...to his house. Because back then, cell phones were limited to the car and were still called car phones. Thus, their love story began on a landline.

Admittedly, Danielle was boy C-R-A-Z-Y back then. Despite her awkward adolescent appearance, she wore her heart on her sleeve. She had braces, untouched eyebrows, and hadn't dated enough to understand that boys like to do the chasing. So, what did she do?

She made a mix tape for him.

She decided to make a music compilation for Bill chocked full of Barenaked Ladies (*"If I had a million dollars I'd buy your love..."*) that would cause him to fall head over heels for her. She was not afraid of his reaction and even had the gumption to call first before appearing at his door.

"Hi, is Bill there?"

"Hello, this is Bill."

"Hi Bill, it's Danielle."

(Pause)

"I made you a mix tape. I'm going to drop it off tonight."

"Uh, okay. Thanks."

"See you soon!"

Romeo and Juliet couldn't have said it better.

As I mentioned, she was only 15 and not capable of driving yet so she had her girlfriend, who had already turned 16, drive her across town to his house. She bravely walked to his front door, rang the doorbell, and handed the tape to his older sister, Erica, who informed Danielle that Bill was not home at the moment. Being a teenage boy, he knew enough to avoid what was presumably going to be a super awkward moment, so he had made himself scarce. But once he came home and found the tape, he knew immediately she was the one he would marry.

Just kidding!

He must have appreciated the gesture just a little, because even though they never really talked about it, a few weeks later, when they were once again at another high school house party, he made "eyes" back at her and it became a classic case of making out and mix tapes; the stuff of teenage dreams. Over the next month, their clandestine affair was her headline news, the type of thing she spent late nights talking about with her girlfriends. Until, like all good things, it had to come to an end when Bill headed off for his freshman year at WVU (Go Mountaineers!). He had one romantic action left in him before their newish relationship fizzled by way of writing her a letter.

With a pen and paper and an envelope with a stamp.

He kept things light and talked about college. Her feelings for him eventually faded, though, as she started her junior year and found another boy to fall madly in love with.

She graduated high school in 1996 and wanted to get the heck out of dodge as fast as she could. Instead of sticking around New York State like most of her pals, Danielle moved to Tempe, Arizona and became an Arizona State University Sun Devil. She became great friends with the girls and guys in her dorm and fully enjoyed the fun that is freshman year as a co-ed. The excitement and good times in Arizona were ephemeral, though. She loved the desert and her new clique of friends out there, but she realized quickly that life at home was moving on without her. By that, I mean our 39-year-old mother gave birth to our little sister Madison that fall, and Danielle was clear across the country.

Quick aside: back then, giving birth at 39 seemed downright crazy, even more so because at the time I was 13 and Danielle was 18. Thankfully Halle Berry and Janet Jackson (can you believe she was 50?!) have since made giving birth at 39 seem like a walk in the park. Amazingly, just a few weeks after delivering Madison, my mom drove with Steve to Phoenix to drop a car off to Danielle so she had a way to get to and from work. That's how tough of a broad our mother is.

After Madison, my mom gave birth to Noah two years later, in 1998. Then the baby train kept on rolling when my father and his wife, Shayne, had Victoria in 1999 and then Andrea (pronounced like Andrea Bocelli, the Italian singer) in 2000.

Four new siblings in four years!

At the time, Danielle and I had no idea that these four kiddos would bless our lives in the most beautiful way. Despite the age gap, having this many siblings has been one of the better things to happen to both of us.

For her upcoming sophomore year, she decided to trade in her cactus and the beautiful vista of Camelback Mountain and set up a life back in Buffalo at the State University of New York at Buffalo (UB) (Go Bulls!) to be closer to home. She was paired with a stranger as a roommate and tried to embrace the bitter winter and her new surroundings. It was a hard transition and one that she did not love. But she was psyched to come home for the summer of 1997 and meet back up with her best friends from high school, three girls all named Kate. What are the odds of that? To add another layer of connectedness, one of the Kates is my husband's older sister. That's true small town living for you.

By this point in time, Danielle had finally come into her own as a young woman. She became the real catch. That summer her hair was sun-kissed and brushed past her shoulders. The braces were long gone and she was no longer lanky. Bill was also home for the summer and had pivoted from a clean-cut all-American boy to the type that followed Phish and the Grateful Dead. Gone were the polos and short hair and in had come longer locks that he could tuck behind his ears. He had gotten contact lenses and exuded the confidence of a college junior.

It was late July and Danielle was volunteering, which she still does to this day, at the annual Italian Festival in town. She had on short jean shorts and a cropped shirt, which, ironically is the style for teeny boppers today. Fashion!

She was working the sausage sandwich line and had noticed a handsome fella stand out in the crowd. Though she ditched her awkward younger self, the boy crazy part had hung on. When Bill, unrecognizable to her with his new 'do and Oakley sunglasses, appeared with money in hand for a sandwich, she felt butterflies.

"Hey Danielle, can I get a sausage sandwich with no peppers and onions?"

For the record, it's the caramelized peppers and onions that marry so well with the sausage that make that sandwich scrumptious. But I digress.

"Sure. But how do you know my name?" She said coyly.

"I'm Bill."

"I'm sorry, but Bill who?"

"Bill Eaton." His invisible tail was immediately now between his legs.

At this moment Danielle turned around to get his veggie-less sandwich and silently made the "wow" face to herself. Cute guy turned out to be Bill Eaton! Imagine that?

Bill took his food and wandered back to his friends. Prior to going over to Danielle's line, Bill had spotted her and told his friends that he was going to make her day. He assumed that she was still impressed with his presence even after all this time.

He was sorely mistaken.

"Guys, she didn't even know who I was," he conceded.

She had kept her eye on him for the remainder of her shift and when it was over, she took off her apron and sauntered over to his group. Her girlfriends had made plans that night to see a concert, Supertramp, about an hour away at a big amusement park. She confidently said to Bill and his crew that they should join them but he rebuffed her offer. His feelings and pride were hurt.

"Oh well," she thought. Bill was not the only fish in her pond that summer. She had another suitor. A tall, dark and handsome Italian boy who was in the military. He was all muscles and he fancied Danielle. They were in the midst of a fun summer fling with no set plans for what was to come. Because unfortunately, at summer's end, he was shipping off to Hawaii for the foreseeable future.

Things became complicated, though, when Bill decided to set his pride aside and spark up a conversation with her when they were both at a bar days later. Their short-lived relationship heated up quite quickly and by early August, they had gone on a few dates. He was heading back to college again but wanted to have one last lunch with her for her birthday, on August 7th. He bought her a WVU t-shirt, that she still has, and asked if she'd come down for the first football game of the season. His fraternity was having a Steak & Champagne formal event at the game and he wanted her to be his date. She weighed the pros and cons of tall, dark, and handsome Italian boy against happy go-lucky Grateful-Dead-loving Bill. Ultimately, she decided that she was magnetically attracted to Bill and couldn't deny the strong connection she had with him.

Bill it was!

After the formal event she attended, they were officially boyfriend and girlfriend. She would make the bi-weekly (and sometimes weekly) four and a half hour treks down to Morgantown, West Virginia from Buffalo. At the time she drove a cherry red Geo Tracker, which I don't believe is even manufactured anymore. It was a small SUV with a soft top roof that looked like it would blow away in a storm if the wind blew too hard. She had outfitted it with cow print seat covers and a bumper sticker that read, "Girls Kick Ass." The tough slogan did not deter thieves, however, from cutting through the soft top and stealing her valuables when she and Bill were once in Camden, New Jersey for a concert.

Danielle would drive down to visit him in rain or snow and always without a mobile device because, again, it was the late 1990s. In that fall semester alone, after they were officially dating, she made the trip 10 whole times. And because it was going so well and she despised life in the Northern Tundra that is Western New York, she transferred down to WVU as soon as she could.

Life went on splendidly for them both, and eventually they moved in together while Danielle was getting her Master's in Education. In 2002, after she graduated, a job opportunity in her current school district popped up, and before they knew it, they were heading back home to plant roots and start a new life. They rented a home directly next to his parents' house before moving into their current home just one house away. They *really* like the West-End street they live on.

Two years later, and after eight years of dating, Bill hatched a plan to propose. Bill made my mom and I aware it was going to happen and we were just giddy with delight at the idea of planning a wedding. Getting hitched was not on Danielle's radar though, not even a little bit. As a child of divorce, she became a non-traditionalist and leaned more towards Goldie Hawn and Oprah's viewpoint on partnership. She figured, if it wasn't broken, why fix it? Eight years of happy times did not have to be interrupted with a wedding. So, one Friday evening in August when Bill appeared before her in a tuxedo as she was skewering veggies onto kabob sticks in advance of a BBQ they were throwing, she was irritated. She was not thinking marriage proposal, she was thinking about marinating meat.

Danielle is the perennial hostess with the mostess and could not be bothered with costumes and pageantry.

"What the heck are you doing?" she asked incredulously.

"Well, you gotta look the part when you ask this serious of a question," he said.

At that moment he dropped to one knee and received the best kiss of his life.

From Truman, the dog.

Truman was nearby and got excited to see his beloved Bill down on his level. He assumed Bill was ready for some quality time with him. Truman's world revolved around Bill, and he took Bill's bended knee as another opportunity to show Bill his affection.

Bill was now the irritated one as he brushed aside the canine and tried to regain composure to get out the most nerve-wracking four words a person can get out.

"Will you marry me?"

She of course said yes as he popped open the ring box. Inside was a stunning solitaire diamond engagement ring in a platinum setting that shone brightly. Relief washed over Bill and he was able to shed the tux for some flip flops. Their impending summer BBQ turned into a lovely engagement celebration with loved ones.

A year later, on August 13, 2005, they had a big, ol' fashioned Italian wedding in front of 300 of their closest friends and family. The bride wore cream, the groom looked dapper once again in a tuxedo, the 5-tiered buttercream cake was adorned with soft pink roses, and everyone drank a little too much.

Ain't love grand?

Their courtship and love story are worth telling because as you've already read, their commitment to one another, in sickness and in health, would be put to the test. Not once, not twice but at least 10 times in seven or so years. Which is where we pick back up. Another hurdle was taking shape.

CHAPTER 7

After the awful night of our brother Noah's graduation in late June of 2016, things never improved. The Sunday that followed was a true struggle for her and she lamented what was to come the following day. On Monday, despite her condition, she had to shuttle her girls to the fun, summer recreation program our city offers to kids once school has ended. The trouble, however, was that Danielle was absolutely in no shape to drive. She still wasn't sleeping and the discomfort had reached a fever pitch. Because of the unending, pulsating pain emanating from her rear end, she was constantly taking Tramadol. And as I mentioned before, she was not comfortable driving while they were in her system. She called for help on this day and asked Bill's father, Gregg, to drive them.

She also placed a call to her GI doctor. She knew it was bad. She knew she needed to be seen and she knew she had reached her breaking point, so much so that on the drive to the rec program, she could only sit on one side of her body because it was too painful to have both butt cheeks flat on the car seat. She clasped the door handle for dear life and let the tears quietly stream down her face so that her carefree daughters in the backseat would not have to see their mom in such despair. Gregg glanced over at Danielle and tears began to well in his eyes too. He put his hand on her shoulder and tried, like Alexis had in D.C., to muster any combination of sympathetic words to make it better.

"It'll be okay. It'll be okay, Danielle."

He fibbed.

Gregg dropped her off back home but she wasn't home long before our mother came and picked her up to take her in to see the GI doctor. Miraculously they had an opening and she could be seen that same day. Another gracious nod to small town living. The only problem was that her actual doctor was still overseas so she was evaluated by his wonderful physician assistant (PA). Though she was an excellent provider, it became a problem only seeing her because she didn't have the authority to make a decision on what to do. While they were discussing the options, Danielle laid down on the examining table and told the PA that she couldn't fight the good fight at home any longer.

"Please, you can't send me home," she pleaded.

Danielle knew that she couldn't suffer any more on her own. Her body was weak and mentally she no longer had the stamina to fight the UC. It was clear that the Remicade infusions were not working and they needed to try something else. She began to cry at the thought of having to pace another night in her living room.

"I can't go on like this. The pain is too much to bear."

The PA agreed completely and leapt into action. She called the GI doc overseas and shared with him how dire of a situation it was and how horrendous Danielle's condition appeared. Her face was drawn and she had no vivacity in her eyes. They agreed she needed to be admitted into the hospital but they couldn't be the ones to make it happen. Technically as a GI doctor, he is considered a consulting physician who does not have the privileges to get her a hospital bed on his own.

But her fantastic primary care doctor did.

The PA called the PCP to see if he'd be willing to admit her sight unseen based on their analysis and he quickly agreed. My mom and Danielle got back in the car and moved fast. Danielle went home to pack a bag and my mom headed for the PCP's office to get the paperwork. Because they had the forms already in hand, once they got to the hospital, they were able to skip registration and were fast-tracked to a room upstairs.

As soon as she arrived in her room, she was given two Norco pain relievers to help her get comfortable. Norco is a brand name for a drug that's comprised of Hydrocodone and Acetaminophen (Tylenol). Again, Danielle allowed her handy dandy white flag of defeat to be flown and a calmness settled in for the first time in weeks. She rejoiced in the fact that she wouldn't have to fight the UC army alone for another minute. Once more, she had reinforcements in the form of IV fluids, nurses to look after her, pain meds to assist with the unmanageable discomfort, and the removal of everyday life stressors.

They also began regularly checking her lab work, which revealed low blood counts once more. This time however, the lower numbers were recorded due to blood loss and poor nutrition. Because her colon was in terrible shape, she was not able to absorb food properly and oftentimes wasn't even hungry. With this hospital stay, the doctors and nurses paid attention to her H&H levels (just a reminder, that stands for hemoglobin and hematocrit).

Here come some more numbers for you to ponder. Although her levels were not off the charts low, they were also not considered normal. On the day of her release from the hospital, they registered her lowest measurements to date:

HGB: **10.5** (the normal range is 12.5 – 16.0 g/dL)

HCT: **31.3** (the normal range is 37.0 – 47.0 %)

Although she had undergone a colonoscopy not that long before, the GI doctor wanted another look. He needed to understand how quickly the disease had progressed and/or if the *C.diff* was back. But this time he knew it was too risky to take the scope all the way up into her colon. He assumed (and rightly so) that her colon was friable and that it could perforate very easily. If you aren't familiar, a perforated bowel is one scary, hot mess to clean up. And I don't mean that in a lighthearted way. It can be a deadly situation if it's not treated and corrected right away. Having stool floating around your system, full of bacteria and the stuff your body is trying to get rid of, is extremely dangerous. Thus, his plan was to do a flexible sigmoidoscopy instead. In layman's terms, that meant he was going to basically just take a peek and not go up into her colon very far. The sigmoid colon is the S-shaped part of the large intestine that resides at the very end and leads into the rectum.

He let her rest on Tuesday (check out the picture she took of herself on this day – she was not ready for her close-up, Mr. DeMille) and on Wednesday the procedure was scheduled. I sound like a broken record but once more, she had the wonderful luck of needing a warm water enema in order for the test to happen. My mom tried from the other side of the door (again) to distract her with banal conversation about anything other than the fact that Danielle was painfully flushing out her system. For Danielle, though, it was just as unbearable as the other instances.

My mom, Steve, and I waited impatiently for her to come back up to her room once the test was over because, though we didn't say it, we collectively knew how big of a moment this was.

They wheeled her into the room and because she had been sedated, she was a little loopy and does not remember waking up and hearing what the results were. Her doctor was a slender man of few words and when he reached the room, he stood in the doorway, in his periwinkle scrubs, to deliver the news. He was kind, but very realistic when he reported his findings to the three of us. It was so serious that when my stepdad, who was working that day and was also in scrubs, went to answer a text message, the GI doctor told him that he needed to focus and pay attention to what he was about to say.

"I confirmed with the test that the UC has gotten worse. It appears the Remicade is not doing the job. It's possible that her body has developed antibodies to fight it. She might have done well initially with it but her body may have responded as if it was a foreign substance that needed to be attacked. We will send her blood sample to a California lab to confirm whether or not that was the case."

(That test cost a mere $3000 to complete and it did prove that her body acted as if the Remicade was a pathogen and developed antibodies to fight it off. Shucks.)

There was a collective sigh from the three of us and

then he continued.

"The next option to try would be the drug Entyvio. It's similar to Remicade and is the next step up the ladder. We need insurance to approve it so we have to get the ball rolling soon."

I believe we asked a few questions and even briefly discussed the possibilities if this new drug didn't work (complete colon removal) but we tried not to get ahead of ourselves. Danielle became more alert after the doctor left and although she was coming off of the medication Versed and wouldn't remember our conversation at all, we filled her in on what the plan was going to be.

In her hazy memory, she has a distinct image of me standing over her with tears in my eyes. It all seemed too much for me to comprehend and as hard as I tried to hide the hopelessness that surrounded her, she could see through my thinly veiled emotions.

We then called Bill as well and shared the news with him while he tied things up at work. With things seemingly okay after everyone knew what the plan was, I left for home. It was around dinner time when I walked in and relieved my little sister from babysitting. But before I could start cooking, my mom called me in a panic.

"Nat, Danielle just spiked a fever of 103 and we asked the ICU doctor on the floor to take a look at her. Maybe you should come back?"

While I had been driving home only minutes before, thinking she was stable and okay, a nurse and co-worker of my mom's had come in to check Danielle's vital signs, something that happens every few hours when you are a patient. Things seemed okay except for her temperature, which had risen very quickly. Fearing the worst (the aforementioned bowel perforation) my mom brought in the intensivist on duty who was nearby at that time. A fringe benefit of working at the hospital was that she had the ability to reach out directly to people who could help if they were available. Danielle's hands were shaking terribly but she was mentally alert.

A CT scan was quickly ordered and executed to rule out a bowel obstruction and possible perforation (a blockage and then rupturing) and when it was confirmed to be negative, they then called back the GI doctor and decided to dose her with antibiotics. They hoped it was just a small instance of the bowel being irritated and emitting a little bit of disease out into her bloodstream. We waited around her bedside and watched as her temperature slowly came back down over time. I headed back home a couple of hours later feeling incredibly forlorn.

I let my thoughts go negative just a bit before putting back on my positive, hopeful, things-will be-okay hat. But in the moment, this is what I was ruminating on:

- Life can be so unfair. She has two, small, adorable girls at home and should be enjoying her summer break.
- Life can also be cut short. Had the seeping infection caused sepsis again, she might not have seen those adorable kids again.
- If the Entyvio doesn't work, what will her life be like without a colon? Does that mean she'd have a colostomy bag and walk around with a pouch of poop attached to her stomach?

Thankfully when I got home, I had my own two, small youngsters to attend to and was able to distract myself with their smiles and not the uncertainty of the future. It was unsettling, though, to leave the hospital, yet another time, and bear witness to a life interrupted due to pain and distress. And there was no guarantee of a concrete cure or a resolution on the horizon.

Since it was approaching the end of June and the July 4th holiday was the following week, my mom, along with her nurse manager, moved mountains on Thursday to get the Entyvio approved, ordered, and hooked up to Danielle via an IV by that Friday; just two days after the sigmoidoscopy — a daunting feat that they overcame extremely quickly. It was a rare event to have it progress that fast but it was surely a cause for a celebration because that meant that we had a plan, we had hope, and we had something in motion that could maybe make her better.

Separately, the question, "what's the plan?" became a common utterance for Danielle. It was quite often during this year that she would call my mom and Steve and ask it. Once they helped her find the answer, she almost immediately felt better, regardless of how discouraging the plan actually was.

Instead of getting an infusion that day, though, Danielle and Bill were *supposed* to be headed down to Pittsburgh (which is about 3 hours away) for a weekend of memorable concert going. They had tickets to see Billy Joel on Friday night and Kenny Chesney on Saturday night. Two of their favorite musicians - all in the same weekend! Just think of the bliss that they were going to incur. We joke as a family that we'd love to come back in our next lives as Bill and Danielle because over the years, they've made a life of attending fabulous concerts.

That particular weekend was supposed to be the start of their freelancing "career" in concert-going. For obvious reasons, they did not go. She was released on Saturday morning and half-heartedly mentioned the Kenny Chesney concert to her GI doctor who didn't think it was a good idea. Both she and Bill were crushed. And mostly because by not going, it meant that her disease was seriously interfering with the fun in their lives.

After she was released from the hospital, my mom and I checked in with her each day (often multiple times) and analyzed every moment of her bathroom routine as if our own lives depended on it. We wondered with desperation if the new medicine was working and scrupulously watched for signs that it was. My mom and I would privately speak (also multiple times) during that same period and hoped this was the magic we'd all been waiting for.

Danielle valiantly tried to attend a wedding on July 9th, just days after being discharged from the hospital, where she pretended to be "normal." The nuptials and reception were held outside at a beautiful, expansive farm. The food was delicious but centered on a true BBQ theme: pulled pork, baked beans served a multitude of ways, corn and other fixins' that would traditionally accompany this type of tasty meal. For Danielle, this provided her with a challenge. Could she successfully eat a greasy, heavy sandwich full of meat and acidic BBQ sauce as well as fiber-rich beans on the side? Could she also try to have a glass of wine like the other guests?

She tried, she really did.

But when her colon decided it was time for her to stop trying, she and Bill had to hightail it home where once more, she found herself needing to hand wash her fancy dress because she didn't beat the clock. This time it was a classic black and white sundress with a sweetheart neckline from the store White House Black Market.

To her credit for braving the wedding, on some days it did seem like the medicine was working and progress was being made. But on other days, it seemed like she was back at the bottom of Mt. Everest staring up at the summit. Thankfully she kept copious notes at that time so she could share them with her doctor and here is what she recorded on July 16th, 2016:

1-3am – *Urges, no stool.*

8am – *Formed, very little blood.*

8:30am – *Looser, very little blood.*

9am – *Raw, formed and little blood.*

9:20am – *Spasm.*

9:45am – *Tylenol, dull throb.*

3:30pm – *Went 2 times. Stool formed. Second time, a little blood.*

9:30pm – *Went 3 times. Last round was painful. Took a Tramadol.*

11:15 – *Absolutely throbbing.*

Midnight – *Took a hot shower.*

1am – *Finally went to bed.*

4am – *Took another Tramadol. Throbbing again.*

And this was a fairly normal 24-hour existence. She even formed a shorthand for herself in describing the symptoms. "S.A.B." meant small amount of blood and "F.D.B." meant few drops of blood. There are a lot of scribbled mentions of medicine taken and hot baths drawn. There were a few accidents noted (once, it happened twice in the same week) and many times the words "throbbing" and "aching" were used. Nowhere in the journal though does she complain that the pain was too much and she couldn't endure any longer. Not a once. She kept things in perspective and tried her darndest to focus on her kids and the life she needed to keep in motion. Frankly, that is a super human achievement if you ask me. Most people would crumble under the weight of living a day in that life let alone the months of it she had to tolerate.

Despite the horrific days she was still living, and the fact that she wasn't sure if the Entyvio was doing its job, Bill and Danielle decided to keep their short vacation with the girls to Presque Isle Beach in Erie, Pennsylvania, as planned from months earlier. Although it's a beach adjacent to Lake Erie, it's a magnificent little slice of heaven for us and it's only 90 minutes away. They had been saving for this jaunt and decided that although her days were by no means perfect, she was "well enough" to give it a go. They packed their bags and headed south for a three-day stay.

The first day was spent at a water park and Danielle did well all things considered. And these were the things that we should all consider: Danielle was at a public water park with a defective and diseased colon and had been hospitalized twice in the last few months because of it. Thus, she was keeping her eye on the bathrooms at all times and was acutely aware that she could have an accident at a moment's notice. She was so aware that she felt anxious about it the whole day. Amazingly, she managed not to poop her pants and was able to give the girls a day of fun without an overtly sick mom.

But as they were departing the park, she implored Bill to drive fast to get to their hotel. She knew she was on borrowed time with regard to having an accident.

"Bill, you might have to stop. I may not make it... Bill, you really might need to stop!"

"It'll be okay Danielle. Can you go a little bit further? We are really close to the hotel if you can hold it a little longer?" He remained calm and tried to put her at ease.

Bill drove as fast as he could to get there. They entered the lobby all together. Danielle impatiently, but politely, asked the front desk agent where the closest bathroom was.

"There is one on the first floor but you have to go down that hall, take a left, then walk down that hallway, and hang a right. It's at the end of that hall by the pool."

Upon hearing that she'd need a map from Lewis & Clark to get to the bathroom, Bill, who had been checking in, slyly handed Danielle the room key as if they were passing a baton in the Olympics. She high-tailed it up there without a thought for their bags or the girls. But she made it. Just barely. And was extremely relieved.

The poop crisis was averted and they all got ready for dinner. Because she felt that she had outsmarted her GI system, she was thrilled for their impending dinner out. Our father is a connoisseur of fantastic restaurants within a three-hour radius of our hometown and had given them a recommendation for a nice Italian place nearby that she was excited to try.

126

Let me just take a second so I can mention our good fortune as children. We were brought up being able to eat out at nice restaurants at least once a week. Because my dad was in the beer business and our local restaurants were his customers, we were lucky enough to enjoy meals out at these establishments on a regular basis. I want to point this out because over the years, a true appreciation for a wonderfully prepared meal, paired with a nice Pinot Noir (for her) and decadent dessert (for me) is something that we both covet and take great pleasure in. So, after a long day at a water park (and an even longer month prior), Danielle was ready to settle into the ambiance and atmosphere of an old-school Italian joint with a fine wine and delicious hand-cut pasta. She was not ready for the goosebumps she got instead.

For some reason, whenever her body began the incessant "urges" to go to the bathroom, which was followed by bloody diarrhea, she would get goosebumps all over her arms first. I do believe there is a medical reason for this which includes nerves to the colon but for the purposes of this story, just know that it was her signal for "drop whatever it is that you're doing and get the hell into the bathroom." The goosebumps arrived right after they sat down and for the duration of their time there, Danielle was ...

Can you guess?

In the bathroom!

She went to the bathroom somewhere between four and six times and was not able to partake in the dinner enjoyment that Bill and the girls had. They paid the bill and headed back to the hotel.

"Bill, why don't you take the girls swimming in the hotel pool and I'll join you as soon as I can."

She hoped that she'd be able to put comfortable clothes on and meet them poolside. Which, if you have kids you already know, is the best part of staying at a hotel for a child - indoor swimming at night. It was such a spectacular time for the girls that May, who was six at the time, learned to swim on her own. But Danielle missed it, and was instead stuck in the hotel bathroom the entire time.

The sun rose the next morning and the hope for a good day streamed into their room. Danielle and Bill had made the decision the night before to play it safe and scrap their morning agenda of lazily lounging on the beach with sand in their toes. They both agreed that if the "urges" appeared, she would not be set up for success (if you know what I mean). They kept their plans, though, to ride on a pirate ship that sailed out on the lake. Bill and the girls braved the open deck while poor Danielle parked her rear end on a cool, metal bench directly next to the bathroom where she stayed for the duration of the voyage. The bench actually felt good based on her pain but she sat there for such a long period of time that the Captain came to check on her because her face screamed, "Dear Lord, please help me to survive the nightmare I'm currently living." Once they became land lubbers again, Bill and Danielle conferred and made the executive decision they needed to go back home and cut their trip one night short.

"What? We can't go home yet! We haven't done the bike ride around the island! You guys said we were going to do that!" Lily argued as best as she could for an eight-year-old.

Danielle gingerly got down on their level in the middle of the hotel parking lot and explained to Lily and May why they were leaving early.

"I'm sorry Lil. I know you were excited about riding our bikes and so was I. I just need a little more time to get better. We will come back, I promise."

On the way back home, Bill and Danielle distracted themselves from their reality and dove back into a conversation they had on their way down to Erie. It involved a magical August trip to the Red Rocks Amphitheatre in Colorado to see Eric Church, a rising country star, perform two nights in a row. As they picked the conversation back up, they knew it was a long shot. They knew she was currently too sick to make that short trip to Erie work. But they sure had fun fantasizing and imagining what it would be like to pause their everyday lives and go across country to see him play. The shows fell around her birthday in early August so they surmised that she'd get another infusion by then and would hopefully be firing on all cylinders at that point. Maybe, just maybe, the plane tickets would be reasonable, the GI doctor would give his blessing, my mom and Steve could babysit, and life as they knew it, would be "normal." The seed was planted in Bill's brain and he was hopeful he could make this happen for Danielle.

After their trip to Erie, Danielle described the pain as a "dull ache" and something she could live with even though her journal entries were still horrific to see. She still went to the bathroom frequently but was able to function to some degree as a mom with kids home for the summer. For the latter half of July, she signed up the girls for a summer enrichment program through our local community college where they went every day from 9:00 in the morning until noon. During those three hours, she had grandiose ideas of all of the gardening and outdoor projects she was going to tackle because she is quite happy with dirt under her fingernails. But what she found was not earthworms and weeds. She found that she didn't have the energy to do anything other than nap during that time. She would drop the girls off, come back home, crawl into bed, and then set an alarm to make sure she was back to pick them up on time.

One instance sticks out in her mind with regard to that enrichment program. She was just about to leave for home after taking the kids into their room when another mom stopped to chat with her. In the middle of their conversation, the goosebumps on her arm appeared and she knew the "urges" were imminent.

"Have you tried that new …?"

"I'm sorry, will you excuse me?" Danielle interrupted abruptly.

She made it to the nearest bathroom and avoided an ugly situation. She was not so fortunate on the way home, though. While driving, in a seated position, her body decided to relieve itself of bloody diarrhea on the nice, tan, leather seat of her new Honda Pilot. She got home and shamefully made her way to the door and had to clean herself and her car before heading back to get them. Clearly, she wasn't improving. She knew it and we knew it. But we all hung our hope on the second infusion which was just days away.

She arrived for the infusion with the weight of

her colon on her shoulders. She needed this dose to work and turn her life around. Since April, life had not been the same. She had endured three straight months of bathroom living. And although she was now a sleuth at finding clean, inconspicuous lavatories, she was ready to poop like a normal person. So, as the medicine infiltrated her system, she prayed all over again.

Bill was also praying. For the medicine to work of course, but also that she'd be better and he could whisk his wife away to Colorado. They had mentioned the trip to my mom and Steve and it wasn't shot down immediately. They understood, with very heavy, empathetic hearts, that Danielle and Bill were both grasping for relief with a side of fun (and beer). They suggested that maybe they pick a different city and a different concert, within driving distance, to try and attend instead of flying across the country. The nature of UC medicine is to knock down one's own immune system a little bit since it's that same system that's essentially attacking itself and causing the colon commotion. But if you remember, the byproduct of that mechanism is that you are more susceptible to colds and infections because your army isn't as strong. Thus, the idea of putting Danielle on a plane with 200 other humans seemed like a hospital stay waiting to happen. Danielle and Bill were steadfast though and basically said, "Colorado or bust!" They heard what my mom and Steve had to say and agreed not to book the tickets for another week. Danielle wanted to speak to her PCP first and see what he had to say about their plan. Luckily, as that week wore on, her symptoms improved. She had one good day, and then another and then another.

In her journal of symptoms, she recorded the following leading up to when they were hoping to leave:

"2-4 bowel movements a day, ache (no Tylenol needed), small amount of blood."

Her symptoms were certainly tolerable and by the time she met with the doctor, he gave his blessing. On one condition.

"Danielle, you have to wear a mask when you are on the plane. We can't risk you getting sick."

(At that time, she would have been the mask-wearing exception. Sadly in 2020 and going forward, that's the rule.)

Yahtzee! They could go. Bill booked the tickets despite the fact that in the week that had passed they had gone up in price. By a lot. You can't put a price tag on joy, though, so he bit the bullet anyway and they were booked for August 9th through the 12th. In preparation for their trip, Danielle purchased not only the face masks but also adult diapers "just in case" an accident occurred. I'm sure it wasn't a proud moment for her but a girl's gotta do what a girl's gotta do.

In booking their trip, they decided to embrace the "when in Rome!" mentality and added an extra day onto the trip on either side. If you're going to fly across country to see not one but two shows by the same artist in the infamous Red Rocks Amphitheatre, why not add extra time to tour a brewery and go tubing down a river? Their plan was to depart very early on Monday morning from Buffalo and return Friday evening with the shows being held Tuesday and Wednesday. Ultimately, their plan became a major travel blessing.

Danielle woke up with the sun at 5:00 to excitedly start her morning routine when she happened to catch a snippet of the news. As she poured her coffee, she began to wonder what airline they were flying as the anchors reported on breaking news regarding airline passengers being stranded at airports all over the country. Since Bill, a closeted travel agent, had booked the trip, she wasn't entirely sure what they were flying until she woke him up for clarification. She gently nudged him awake and asked which carrier he had gone with.

"Delta. Why?"

"Uh oh. Houston, we have a problem. You better come see this."

Apparently, Delta's main computer system went down and it caused absolute chaos for every passenger holding a Delta ticket for that day, in the U.S. and across the world. After waiting in dreadfully long lines at the Buffalo airport, they were routed to Detroit with a departure for Denver TBD. They figured some movement was better than none and boarded the plane. When they arrived around 11:00 at night, tired and bummed not to be at their final destination, they were greeted with more unfortunate news. They were not leaving for Colorado until the next morning. And because Delta was now having to accommodate thousands of other stranded passengers, they were going to receive a lodging voucher for a small motel, in a run-down part of town, 45 minutes away from the airport. Danielle and Bill were good sports through it all, knowing they were blessed to even be taking the trip.

They had to be back at the airport the next morning at the ripe hour of 4:00 so they did not sleep much. Danielle was still figuring out her bathroom routine and how her body responded to different foods so it was not an ideal situation but they made the best of the short time they were in Detroit Motor City. Eventually they did get out of there and made it to their much nicer hotel in Golden, Colorado with just enough time to join their scheduled Coors' Brewery tour and then on to the show. Though they were exhausted, night number one was a total success. No issues, no urges, no pain! It was an Eric Church "Drink in My Hand" miracle.

Concert number one gave her confidence and it gave her hope that she could lead a normal life once more. With day number two upon them and the extra pep in her step, they decided to consult maps and ask some locals where they could find a good hiking trail nearby. They were currently surrounded by Colorado's prized possession, the Rocky Mountains, and they figured they better seize the opportunity to explore something magnificent so off they went.

With each step Danielle took, she contemplated the summer she had just experienced and was eternally grateful to bear witness to her present surroundings. She took it nice and easy and even let Bill go ahead a bit so that she could take it all in, at her own pace. The air was thinner and drier and she didn't want to over exert herself in an unfamiliar place. Yet, she was brave. And she was also extremely aware that she was in between the sick life she despised and the healthy life for which she wanted to return. The hike only lasted a few hours but it was a symbolic moment for her and one that has been embedded in her memory ever since. She had escaped the bowels of hell (pun intended) and was close enough to heaven that she could almost reach up and touch it. She fully understood what this hike meant and was not going to waste it.

Reality set back in before the show on that second night. While she was getting ready and Bill was in the bathroom, she had a strong, all-hands-on-deck type of urge to use the bathroom, right then and right there.

"Bill! I need to get in there and I need to do it right now," she yelled.

He understood immediately and hopped out as soon as he could. Fearing the worst, Danielle donned her Depends before they headed out and prayed for another break to what her life had become over the last few months.

It is the exact reason listed above (the fact that a 38-year-old woman was wearing Depends to a concert at Red Rocks) that she and Bill relied on when they threw caution to the wind and bought fifth row seats in the center of the ampitheatre for night number two. Go big or go home... with your Depends!

Before she settled into her seat with the luxurious fifth row view, Danielle did what she had gotten in the habit of doing when out in public, mapping out the safest and easiest bathroom. She consulted a really nice security guard who gave her a wonderful gift.

"Well, if you look in that direction, you'll see a women's restroom that's close, which is why the line is extremely long. However, there's also a women's bathroom that's just off to the right and down a few steps. It seems like it's a secret because it's out of the way but it's really not, so feel free to use it. Most people just don't even know it's there," he shared.

Yeehaw!

"Thank you very much!" she said with true gratitude.

With that glorious knowledge in her back pocket, Danielle was able to enjoy her suds like a normal(ish) person for the rest of the night.

Because they were so close to the Coors' Factory, the only type of beer the amphitheatre sold was Coors Original (a.k.a. Banquet Beer for those of us who have a strong connection to the brand). Danielle tempted fate a little bit by having four ice cold cups in honor of our family's ties with the Coors' family, which do run strong. For example, during my family's 100th anniversary celebration of being in the beer business back in 2012, Pete Coors flew to our warehouse to be a part of the festivities. So, to say that Danielle fully appreciated her pints would be an understatement.

In the back of her head, she worried, though. In general, four beers are a lot for her to consume but especially given her sensitive GI tract. Would this come back to haunt her in the wee hours of the morning? Thankfully, the universe gave her a pass on this night. It wouldn't always, but on this night, she was able to drink her beer and enjoy it too.

Before they left Golden for Denver, they rented tubes for a magical tubing adventure down Clear Creek, the same body of water that flows into the Coors Brewery. The water lived up to its name, it was crystal clear and rushed over the smooth river rocks at the perfect speed for tubing. In the warm August sun, they slowly meandered down the waterway with breathtaking views all around them. It felt like paradise and it allowed them both to be relaxed and carefree.

Once they reached the end of the river, they found their way to their rental car and headed into Denver for their hipster, boutique hotel for one more night away. It was equipped with a fantastic patio and a gorgeous bathroom, a space that Danielle appreciated to the fullest. Though they were not in town long, they enjoyed themselves immensely. During their downtime in the hotel room, Danielle luxuriously reclined in the sitting area and read a book – without any interruptions and without tremendous pain. A first for her in a long while.

Danielle also made sure there was time in the itinerary for some shopping. And shop she did. So much so that our family still talks about the bathing suit she purchased on this trip. She bought a three-piece Nanette Lepore suit, with a beautiful pink paisley print, for $300.

Three hundred dollars!

To J. Lo or Julia Roberts I'm sure that would be a bargain but for an 8th grade history teacher from Western New York, she should be wearing that bathing suit everywhere she goes. And then twice on Sundays. She still has it thankfully and made zero apologies for the purchase after everything she had been through. Despite poor Bill almost having a minor heart attack when he heard the sales associate say, "That comes to 300 hundred dollars even." It fit her like a glove and that was that. She was also a patron of "the most marvelous Banana Republic store" she had ever seen where she bought a pair of tight-fitting jeans she wears when she wants to get gussied up. Every time she wears them, she remembers the bliss she had in her heart when they were on that trip. A nice reminder of how you can go through something tough, and still find joy and fun, even if you have to fly across the country to get it.

Overall, that trip was the best prescription she could have been given. It rejuvenated them both and gave them the strength to keep on going, literally.

Earlier in the year, before their life became solely about Danielle's large intestine, they had also planned a fun-filled RV trip (without the girls) surrounding a Jimmy Buffett concert in Pittsburgh at the end of August. Now that they were home from Colorado, the Buffett trip was upon them. Along with his parents, Bill's brother and his aunt, they meet every year for a weekend of music and Parrot Head jubilation. If you haven't been to a Buffett show in your life, it's worth it. There's a camaraderie amongst the fans that I would liken to a fraternity or sorority. Your fellow concert goers (after a little alcohol) become like family because the tailgating at these shows could be an Olympic sport. There's dancing, women in coconut bras, men doing keg stands, beer pong, hot dogs on portable grills, and "Cheeseburger in Paradise" on repeat. It's a sight to see. So much so that during Jimmy's set, he uses video footage that his team captures from the tailgating shenanigans in each city to play in the background of his set.

She had received another Entyvio injection before they left for Pittsburgh and everyone was still hoping this medication was going to be her salvation. She wasn't 100 percent better, but she was getting by. She even had the time and energy to prepare a beautiful platter of garden-fresh bruschetta for the ride down in the RV. Her bruschetta is a magical combination of soft goat cheese spread on crusty baguette slices topped with chopped grape tomatoes, basil, and toasted pine nuts. She made it, packed it up, and ate it as they headed down south in the newly purchased but well-loved 1980s-era RV that Gregg and Rhonda now owned as a retired couple. It wasn't the flashiest of recreational vehicles but it provided them with all the necessary amenities for a trip like this.

If you are an Eaton and you are in road trip mode, your goal is to get where you're going as fast as possible with the fewest number of stops. Thus, the RV was a great vehicle to travel in. True to form, though, when they made a quick pit stop at an outlet mall halfway down, Danielle promised she was only running into one store to buy a nice school planner for the impending year. However, her fashion sense was triggered when she briskly walked by the Tommy Hilfiger outlet store and eyed two stunning and must-have dresses perfect for autumn. Pawnee's own Donna Meagle exclaiming, "Treat yo-self," ran through her mind and in seven minutes or less she tried on, admired, and purchased the two gorgeous frocks *plus* she had time to snag the planner.

They made it down to Pittsburgh safe and sound and Danielle's journal entry from that travel day doesn't look too awful. However, the following day, the day of the show, was not pleasant.

> *Up 2-3 times to pee in the night with gas and bright red blood.*
> **8am** – *Stool, S.A.B.* (small amount of blood)
> **8:15am** – *Attempt, ashy-colored stool.*
> **9am** – *Stool, S.A.B. at breakfast. Dull ache* intensified.
> **10:30am** – *Urgent, small amount of stool, blood.*
> **(Concert – tailgating – drinking – ate bruschetta)**
> **Midnight** – *Stool, bright red blood, terrible ache, took Tramadol.*

12:15am – *Again, stool, bright red blood, terrible ache.*
12:20am – *Spasm.*
6am – *Gas, bright red blood, ache.*

That morning at breakfast, Bill's father noticed something was off with Danielle as she got up from sitting and had to pace around the hotel's breakfast room.

"Danielle, is everything okay?" he wondered.

"Yes, we've just been sitting here awhile waiting for our food." She was telling the truth but was also telling a white lie. She was fully engulfed in the aching rear-end that was causing her to pace.

It wasn't the horrific pain she'd experienced before, but it was definitely there. Think about having a pebble in your shoe. You feel it, you know it's there every time you take a step, but it's not a rusty nail so you can keep going. That's what she was feeling on this morning. As she retraced her eating habits from the day before she tried to come up with a reason. She had eaten those tomatoes on the bruschetta and maybe the acid and the seeds were giving her trouble? She couldn't be totally sure but hoped that if she avoided acidic foods and all types of wine for the next week, she'd probably be fine. She convinced herself that the medicine had been working and this was just a case of her needing to truly respect her diet and not indulge like someone could with normal anatomy.

I'll mail you a dollar if you can guess what I'm about to say, though?

Unfortunately, Danielle was wrong. It wasn't about the tomato seeds or the beers she had while she was wasting away in Margaritaville.

The Entyvio stopped working. It had failed as well. She didn't know it yet but she was essentially out of medicinal options.

CHAPTER 8

One day after returning home from the Buffett concert, Danielle was set to go back to school for two days, Thursday and Friday. Working these two days were part of her union contract and included in-services and meetings without students. Instead of planning lessons, tweaking PowerPoints and coordinating her fabulous outfits in the hours she had before it was back to work, Danielle found herself in the same position she had been in many, many times before. She was wishing and hoping her situation would improve so she could do what she normally did on any given day. She went to bed hoping for a good night but was up every hour with urges and discomfort that caused her to break down and take a Tramadol. She viewed taking the medicine as a defeat because she knew it would leave her feeling groggy for that first day. She dug deep and found the energy to get dressed, put on some make up and head into school like she normally would. It didn't help her cause, though, that part of the presentation she was sitting in on had her standing up and sitting down frequently. A good feature for someone wanting to stay active while sitting but bad for someone with a tender bottom. She wondered how she was going to get through the whole day in the shape she was presently in.

Across the room she spotted a new member of her 8th grade teaching team, the science teacher. Normally she would have made the time to seek her out and provide a warm and friendly welcome. Today though, Danielle had no oomph. She could not find the strength to be cheerful and hospitable to her new co-worker. She just did not have it in her.

She tried again the next day to put one foot in front of the other and make herself be the productive school employee she normally exemplified but she was unsuccessful. She surrendered around lunchtime and knew she needed help in general but in the immediate moment, needed to get home.

In a funny twist of fate, Danielle was assigned a new teacher's assistant for this upcoming year. She had never had someone work in her room before but she was blessed to be paired with my husband Mike's Aunt Julie. Julie is kind, excellent at organization, and provides an unspoken air of helpfulness. She always thinks two steps ahead and is prepared for something even when you didn't realize you needed to be prepared.

Five years before this encounter, Julie suffered the unspeakable tragedy of losing her daughter, Mike's cousin Andrea, at the age of 21, just four weeks after her milestone birthday. Andrea was attending Ithaca College as a student of their DPT (Doctor of Physical Therapy) program with a minor in Business. It was a six-year program and she was almost done with her third year. The summer prior to her passing she had completed a mini-study abroad program in Beijing, China where she learned their physical therapy and acupuncture methods. Aside from being incredibly smart, she was also a gifted singer and had an ebullient personality.

But sometimes the universe works in mysterious

ways. When she was renewing her driver's license after turning 21, Andrea made the noble decision, after talking with Julie first, to become an organ donor.

Then she got sick with mononucleosis.

Shockingly, Andrea succumbed to complications from having mono and died on April 29th, 2009.

The mono had spread through her body and was affecting the alveoli (the tiny air sacs that help with oxygen exchange) in her lungs. She needed routine breathing assistance to help fight it off which put her in the hospital. The doctors attended to her all night to provide her with the necessary breathing treatments she needed. Then, the following day, after being admitted, it was decided she should be intubated for easier breathing; something that should have been a quick process to help her heal and recover. Unfortunately, that is not what occurred. After she was anesthetized, they put the intubation tube into her esophagus, not into her trachea where it should have been. Andrea was without oxygen for 20 long minutes. As a result, she went into cardiac arrest on the operating table. She was kept alive via machines but died a few days later, ultimately from oxygen deprivation to her brain. Her death became an enormous case of medical malpractice that could have been prevented entirely.

Her very untimely passing left her mom, her father Rich and her siblings Brittney and Eric, to try and live on without her. Because of that awful heartbreak that no parent should ever endure, and in spite of it, Julie's compassion and empathy for others grew exponentially.

So, that day at lunch when Danielle was packing up to leave early, she didn't realize the ally she would have in Julie as time went on.

Danielle briefly explained her situation.

"I'm not sure if you know this Julie, but I have this disease, ulcerative colitis, and right now, I'm struggling. I'm really in bad shape. I don't know what's going to happen but I think I'll be out of school for a while."

Tears welled in both of their eyes and Danielle's voiced cracked as she said goodbye.

Julie absorbed what Danielle had to say and although they hadn't worked together before, was able to jump in and help secure a substitute for her. Danielle had left her lesson plans for the substitute and walked out of the school unsure of what was going to happen. She knew trouble was lurking for her and that surgery may be in her future but the extent of what was to happen was unfathomable.

Tired, sore and losing her grasp on her life once more, Danielle made another desperate call to see her GI doctor for some answers on what the next steps could be. The appointment happened shortly thereafter. She sat on the examining table and he chose his words carefully because he knew he was delivering a major blow to Danielle's confidence.

"I believe we have reached the end of the road as far as my services go. I can't help you any longer so you have a choice to make. I can refer you to a new group of providers in Rochester or the Cleveland Clinic who would be better acquainted with cases like yours. We could try Humira but because your body has rejected the other two biologics, I don't feel that you would respond well. And that would just prolong your discomfort and pain."

For Danielle, at that moment, all of the sunshine in the room vanished.

Her doctor was intelligent, helpful, and for five years had been her resource for all of the ups and downs she had experienced. And now, he was telling her he had no more tricks up his sleeve. He had officially run out of options and alternatives to help her.

Danielle had gone to that appointment by herself and was forced to sit with this life-altering news alone, which left her feeling petrified. A month or so before, when she was in his office, she had asked if he could recommend surgery so that her troubles could magically go away. And at that time her doctor was somber and extremely serious in his response.

"Danielle, that is not a path you want to go down unless we've completely run out of options. It's a very serious process with the potential for many complications."

Thus, the magnitude of what he was presently saying hit her like a ton of bricks. And not even the red clay kind. She was struck to her core with massive concrete blocks.

She was most likely heading down the avenue he explicitly wanted to avoid just a short time ago. She wondered how could she manage something so serious with a full-time job and a young family.

She chose to move forward with Rochester because the Cleveland Clinic is three and a half hours away, although Rochester is not close either. For anyone not well-versed in the geography of Western New York, Rochester is an hour and 45 minutes northeast of Olean. It is not the easiest commute when you have to be near a bathroom at all times and cannot sit for long periods of time but it was still closer.

She was at the mercy of her new provider's office to reach out to make a new appointment so she filled her days with rest until Rochester finally called. Thankfully she only had to wait a week before she could be seen.

She and my mom drove up together for a morning appointment with the new GI specialist. He was an older gentleman who turned out to be...

The wrong guy.

Somewhere along the way, a disconnect occurred between Danielle and this man who was about to retire and who focused on patients with Crohn's instead of UC. Just when they both wanted to toss their arms up in frustration, they were able to snag an afternoon appointment with another provider in the same group who was more appropriate for Danielle's case. They had a few hours to waste before they were able to get in so they went and had lunch nearby and strolled through a Barnes & Noble around the corner from the hospital complex. I remember calling my mom that day to check on their progress and to get an update.

"How's she holding up?" I inquired.

"Well, she's really tired. She's used to napping every day and she's not able to do that right now so she's sitting in a comfy chair here in Barnes & Noble. She looks absolutely exhausted. But hopefully we get some answers from this other guy. Cross your fingers."

My mom held up a good front that day for Danielle but I know she was scared. We all knew that she was headed for surgery and the risks and complications that went along with that type of intervention seemed so much worse that what she was currently dealing with. Yet, we still said our prayers and hoped the new doctor had good news.

He ended up being a very smart physician who was all business. He had gotten the scoop from his PA and came in ready to tackle the problem.

"Good afternoon. It seems that we have two options based on your history. We can try the Humira and see if it works or we can plan for the surgery."

While Danielle was processing her choices, my mom took the reins.

"Doctor, if this was your daughter, what would you do?"

"I would move forward with the surgery."

Once they made the decision, things moved fairly quickly. He scheduled her for the following day to meet with the surgeon and planned for more tests to be conducted the following week. She needed more blood work drawn, another colonoscopy, and an MRI of her belly. Though it wasn't great news, it was a small semblance of a plan and Danielle grabbed onto it tightly. We all had many questions that we hoped to find answers to the following day when they met with the actual surgeon.

Bill took the day off and drove her because she not only had to see the surgeon at 3:00 but was also set for the MRI afterward, at 4:45. They did not wait long before meeting with the surgical PA. She listened to their story and took notes before handing it off to the surgeon. They had no pre-conceived notions about the surgeon other than she was a woman and she had an Italian last name.

When she walked in, she set a more resolute tone for how most of their interactions would be for the next year. She arrived not in scrubs but in a stunning black and white wrap dress that fit her lean frame impeccably. Her ensemble was accentuated with a pair of trendy black kitten heels. Her dark brown hair was styled flawlessly, giving her the appearance of a kick-ass surgeon you'd see on *Grey's Anatomy*. Though she didn't mince any words in her explanation, she gave them both the gift of time — a rarity for the norm in healthcare today. Over the course of an hour, the surgeon walked them through every single step of the process using diagrams and drawings so they knew exactly what was coming and the grave risks associated with each step. Her explanation resembled the following:

- The formal name of the total procedure is the tongue twisting title, "proctocolectomy with ileal pouch anal-anastomosis." Its acronym is also used, IPAA, but for the most part, people use a colloquialism, J-pouch, more frequently.
- Her doctor would conduct three surgeries on Danielle, with the help of a robotic arm, spread over a year's time. After each procedure, her body would need to recover for at least eight weeks before the next surgery could be scheduled.
- The first surgery would remove her original large intestine almost completely all the way down to the base of her rectum. They would then give her an ostomy bag that she would live with for ten months.
- The second surgery's purpose was to create

the "J-pouch" (her future new "large" intestine). They would use part of her small intestine to create what looks like a "J." It wouldn't be connected at that time because her body needed time to rest and heal (so that stool wasn't passing through the new parts). The surgeon also stated that this surgery would leave her feeling pretty rotten. Danielle would come to the operating table feeling fairly well and would be left feeling lousy. Unlike the first surgery where she'd come to them desperate for relief from the illness and finding it with the removal of the diseased organ.

- The third and last procedure would take away the ostomy bag and formally hook up the J-pouch to her rectum so her stool could flow through her body in a more normal way.

- Once fully healed, her new normal would not represent what's normal to someone with both intestines. She would still need to go to the bathroom somewhere between eight and twelve times. Everyday. Including when she was at work. She would also need to keep herself hydrated extremely well and still monitor her diet to help prevent going number two even more frequently than the eight to twelve times she should expect.

- She was also given a lifetime permission slip to eat as many potato chips as humanly possible because of their high level of sodium. Because her GI tract would become a lot shorter, food would move through it rather quickly. As a result, her body would not retain water like it should. Sodium helps counteract that facet of her life post-surgery. To assist with this consequence, she was also told

to consume lots and lots of liquids. Forever and for always. She would become someone that has to drink as much fluid as possible each and every day.
- As for the risks and complications, the surgeon discussed several. They ranged in the level severity but for the most part they all fell into the terrifying category.

"In looking at the possible negative outcomes with the third surgery, there is a chance you could have anal leakage (eek, my word). Your body could also reject the new pouch we will create for you and you'd have to live with the external ostomy permanently. There is also a very small chance that even after we remove the diseased colon, your body will adapt and begin attacking other portions of your GI tract, which in essence becomes Crohn's. But that is not is something to spend time worrying about."

Danielle took it all in and was visibly surprised by the gravity of what was before her. Her mouth hung open as she mentally pictured what the next twelve months would consist of: three massive surgeries that would take place almost two hours away from home. Plus, they were given the first procedure date, September 22nd, 2016, which made it all very concrete. Her new plan involved a date in the near future where a major organ of hers would be removed.

Holy cannoli, Batman!

Once the appointment with the surgeon was over, she had to go directly to get an MRI scan of her belly. MRIs are not peaceful or calming in any way – the antithesis of what she needed to experience after digesting the granular details of having pieces of her anatomy removed and repurposed. So, by the time Danielle set foot into the nuclear medicine department, she became emotionally unhinged. A cavern of desolation had formed within her. She began to ugly cry and couldn't pull herself together. She started to speak to the radiology techs but had to pull back on what she was saying because she was truly hysterical. It took a few minutes but eventually the unrelenting tears subsided and she was able to lie down and withstand the jarring and lengthy circumstance that is an MRI.

After a tiresome day full of distress and sadness, not to mention the consistent pain and frequent bathroom trips that she still had to contend with, Bill and Danielle finally got into their car around 7:00 that night. Bill hadn't even shifted into drive before the emotions bubbled to the surface for Danielle once again. Danielle felt sorrow and anguish unlike anything she could formally put into words.

"Bill, how am I going to do this? I can't go through with it," she wailed.

He tried to dial into his eternal well of optimism.

"It will be okay. You can do it. This is going to help you."

At that point, Danielle became angry with him.

How could he be so positive after hearing that she'd have to live with a bag of poop attached to her stomach for TEN whole months!

"Bill, I just turned 38! This is not how it's supposed to be. No one my age should have to worry about emptying a pouch of stool a few times a day. How can I start and stop being a teacher to my students three separate times throughout the school year? How will Lily and May be affected by me being away in a hospital? How can I take care of them while I'm recuperating?"

Bill became frustrated then.

"Danielle, do you remember the surgeon saying that if you didn't go through with this, you'd most likely end up with colon cancer? The facts are there. People with UC are at a greater risk of developing it. We need you around. Our girls need you around. We don't need you getting colon cancer! This will eliminate that threat from our lives. You have to do it."

[In 2020, according to the American Cancer Society, excluding skin cancers, colorectal cancer is the third most common cancer diagnosed in both men and women here in the United States. And the number is rising for those under 50 who are diagnosed with it.]

The tears then started to flow for Bill and they were both sobbing in the parking lot.

Bill collected himself after a few minutes and was eventually able to put the car in drive. The long ride home was a solemn one for them both.

I was at their house that night babysitting the girls because it was a school night and they needed to get to bed at a reasonable time. I had a million and one questions about their day but when they got home, I could feel the dreariness hovering over each of them. It wasn't the time to pepper them with my inquiries so I tried to respect their feelings and scoot out of there as fast as I could. They both looked like lost puppies seeking salvation.

The following Monday rolled around and Danielle

was scheduled to be in Rochester that afternoon for her colonoscopy. Although her new GI doctor and the surgeon could view the images from her summer colonoscopy, they wanted one last clear picture of what they were up against and how far the disease had spread. Danielle was supposed to follow a colonoscopy protocol on Sunday that involved A LOT of MiraLAX. However, in her exhausted state, she misunderstood the amount she was supposed to consume and had to double up on it that morning. Which meant that on the ride up to the hospital, she and my mom had to stop a few times so she could use the restroom and evacuate what was left in her colon. They made it to a small town where there was an ALDI grocery store and she used the facilities there not once, not twice, but three times. Each time she thought she was done but by the time she got out to the car she had to run right back in and go some more.

Before they stopped, with white knuckles gripping the door handle, she prayed hard to the God of Sphincters because she was not sure she'd make it and thought she might have an accident in my mom's nice, new Toyota 4Runner. She had kindly thought ahead and had towels all around the seat she was sitting in but still, no grown adult wants to poop in their parent's car.

Because of her MiraLAX misunderstanding, she was worried she wouldn't be cleared for the test and that day would be useless. That little worry snowballed into a greater worry that if the colonoscopy appointment would have to be pushed back, then so would the surgery date. And that would push back the other two surgery dates and that meant more time out of work for her. It was important for her as a working professional. But more importantly, her worries increased in intensity at the thought of her students being without their history teacher so much that year. She teaches in a high-poverty area, and school can sometimes be the most stable place for her kids, a fact not lost on Danielle or any other teacher there. She thought of her students and how her error could cost them some much-needed stability.

I happened to be down in Atlanta that day on a work trip. I was in a long meeting but stepped out to touch base with my mom. She gave me the run-down and the pit in my stomach for my sister grew bigger. Here I was on an all-expenses paid trip down South, eating a delicious take-out lunch from California Pizza Kitchen, in a fancy boardroom, while my sister was in a grocery store bathroom relieving herself uncontrollably.

In spite of it all, she survived the ride and was able to get the scope.

Phew!

It proved what we all knew: Her new doctor described her colon as "kaput and colorless." It was coming out for sure and the September 22nd removal date could not come soon enough for her.

Although the time in between waiting and the surgery was not without stress.

One Sunday evening before the first surgery, Danielle, Bill, and the kids went down to his parents' house for a cookout, a tradition Rhonda liked to honor as much as she could. She has a big, welcoming dining room table that could seat 12 people comfortably and she liked to fill it with her family as much as possible. She's a wonderful hostess and a darn good cook. At Christmas she's known for hot ham and cheese sandwiches wrapped in tin foil to be eaten by the handful. On this night, they were all sitting around the table eating hot dogs and hamburgers when in the middle of chewing, Danielle put her hands up to her face and began to cry. She was trying to follow the conversation happening in front of her, but her mind was focused on the impending, life-altering surgery coming up.

There was a collective conversational pause by everyone in the group while they watched Danielle sob into her macaroni salad. Everyone took a beat and let her have a moment. Everyone except for Bill's younger brother, Gregory, who stepped up to the plate. Normally Gregory is a quick-witted jokester but, at this meal, in that moment, he summoned the perfect things to say.

"Danielle, you will be okay. We know how hard this is for you but you are a strong person and we will all be here for you, Bill, and the girls. Whenever and wherever you need it."

It didn't take away the internal strife she was experiencing but it was clear evidence of the team of supporters that Danielle had in her corner.

A few days before the big day, Danielle, along with my mom and Steve, went back up to Rochester to meet with two special and kind people that would help her mentally and physically throughout this part of her UC journey, the Ostomy Center Program Director & Nurse Practitioner (NP), and an Ostomy Center volunteer.

Meeting with the NP was a vital step in the process because her purpose was to teach Danielle about caring for and cleaning her bag, what her skin should look like, the tools to use, and what types of issues to watch out for. She is one of the only NPs in the area who specializes in complex dermatological issues related to ostomy bag care so she had an unmatched cache of knowledge. Because of the dearth of information she was tasked with communicating, Danielle's eyes were opened to an overwhelming amount of content. She stuck to the science of what was going to happen and broke down the specifics. It became a long appointment because they needed to mark her belly with permanent marker to let the surgeon know where the bag should go. They also tested spots based on where Danielle wears her pants so that the waistband didn't rub up against it and cause damage or allow the bag to become unattached.

She was also extremely kind throughout the appointment and going forward was always there for Danielle as she moved through each surgery. She made herself available for questions or follow-up appointments even when it seemed that she didn't really have the time. Danielle was truly blessed to have been placed in her care. Being a specialized provider like this NP can be a tough job, but she answered her call of duty with grace and professionalism, always putting her patients first.

Once the NP was finished with her portion of the appointment, the center volunteer, a vivacious woman in her seventies, came in to talk to Danielle about the logistics and the emotional side of everyday life with an ostomy bag.

This woman also holds a special place in Danielle's heart. She was an excellent resource for Danielle throughout her ordeal in addition to being extremely sympathetic and kind. To this day, they still send one another

Christmas cards.

Before the volunteer even spoke a word during their first meeting, Danielle broke down in tears. She had done an excellent job holding it together while the NP spoke but here was a living, breathing woman she could reach out and touch that was living and breathing with something Danielle was about to be given. The weight of the moment struck her and she just sobbed.

Thankfully, this volunteer was the perfect match for Danielle because she had been living with an ostomy bag for many years and was content to keep it that way until the day she died. Her friendly demeanor and casual discussion on the ins and outs of having one quickly made Danielle feel more comfortable and even allowed her to crack a smile when she wanted to play a game.

"Okay everyone. Who in this room is living with an ostomy bag? Can you tell I have one? I bet you can't!"

As she spoke, she twirled around showing off the skin tight jeans and sweater she was wearing. They all agreed she looked fabulous and would have never been able to tell her secret from what they could see. It really eased the mood in the room.

Then she mentioned s-e-x.

The room they were crammed into was tiny. About the size of an exam room in a pediatrician's office. It was not necessarily meant for an NP, the volunteer, Danielle *and* my mom and Steve, who were still present. So, when the volunteer began asking how active she and Bill's sex life was and how that would be affected, the tiny room seemed to close in on Danielle. She blushed in a way only a Catholic girl can.

When we were kids, we did not, under any uncertain terms, discuss the parts of one's body that exists "between your legs." If you needed to reference that area for some reason, that's what you said. For example, while taking a bath as a child you'd say, "Yes mom, I washed between my legs." If you ever heard our mother discussing s-e-x, she called it "fooling around." When our father gave Danielle the birds and bees discussion at dinner one night, it was so painful that she thought it would be more pleasurable to dig her fork into her leg really hard. She figured (and hoped) that her leg pain would take away from the incoming infiltration of audible pain she was about to experience.

The same fear and anxiety rushed to her head as the volunteer waited for an answer. Thankfully, Danielle was able to switch the subject before she passed out. She remembers that extremely awkward moment as horrifying. (Sorry Danielle, it's a little funny, though, all these years later).

C'mon, who doesn't love talking about being sexually intimate with your husband while your mother, stepfather, and two strangers listen in on the juicy details?

CHAPTER 9

Finally, the surgery day was upon them. It was a pretty Thursday morning in Autumn that Danielle could not appreciate because she was, in unpoetic millennial terms, a hot mess. She did not sleep well the night before and cried the entire way up to the hospital. My mom and Steve drove up in one car while Bill and Danielle were in another. While they were driving, my mom called Danielle to check in and Danielle couldn't speak. She was scared to death. Her biggest fear was that she wasn't going to wake up and her kids would be left without a mother. A fact that no one, not even Steve as a physician, could promise wouldn't happen with 100 percent total certainly. It wasn't a likely scenario, but awful things can occur in an operating room. We've all seen *ER* and the aforementioned *Grey's Anatomy*. And that's why those scripted medical dramas garner such high ratings. Things can go sideways rather quickly. So, until the moment when she was forced to leave them, her hands were clutching onto Bill and my mom so very tightly. It wasn't until the anesthesiologist put the mask over her mouth and nose and had her begin counting backwards did she finally let go. Before submitting to the anesthesia drugs, she remembers hearing classic rock tunes in the background. It would be her surgeon's choice for all three surgeries and it made Danielle feel at ease. We grew up listening to our rock 'n roll-loving father playing Led

Zeppelin, The Who, Pink Floyd and other great artists of that era on his record player. To Danielle, this was a good omen.

The surgery was extensive and lasted four hours. They told her it would be the longest of the three. My mom, Bill and Steve tried to pass the time in the busy lobby area by reading the paper, grabbing lunch, and talking to family members. But when you are focused on making sure someone survives, it feels like an eternity to be kept waiting. They received calls from the operating room just about every hour letting them know she was doing okay.

Back in Olean, I was a nervous wreck. My son Sawyer was only one at the time and Sadie was three. I had made the decision to step away from working full time to be home with them, so I wasn't able to be there. And it was difficult. I knew my mom would keep me posted, but it was impossible to focus on anything other than the fact that Danielle was having major abdominal surgery.

The final call came and Bill was assured that she had done well and was headed up to the floor where she would be spending the next few days. They had to wait a little longer for Danielle to get settled in but then they were all allowed to go visit her.

When Danielle's eyes opened in the recovery room, she was relieved but still petrified. She began to cry immediately and wanted to see her people. She was genuinely happy to be alive but was experiencing sensations and pain unlike anything she had dealt with before.

If you are eating your cheerios while reading this, you may want to set them aside for a moment while I briefly describe what occurs in order to hook up an ostomy bag.

Because she was now without a large intestine, they took the end of her small intestine and brought it up and out of her belly (just a smidge) so it could connect to the ostomy bag parts. This is called a stoma. Picture a hole at the top right of your stomach where there's a piece of intestine protruding out. Because the stoma was new, the site was swollen and grotesque. It was bulbous in nature and because it was technically still her intestine, it wiggled on its own. Overall, it was very painful and left Danielle with a completely foreign feeling. She was also told at this time that a very small piece of her large intestine, a stump, had been left attached to her rectum so that during the 3rd surgery there would be some connective tissue they could use when the new J-pouch would be affixed. Although this stump was extremely small, just centimeters in length, they warned her that it could still be diseased and could cause her to have the same issues she's had all along, pain and bloody stools.

Which of course it did.

That stinkin' stump fought her until the bitter end. She was able to give herself enemas to combat those symptoms but it was still a fantastic addition on top of the other things she had to pay attention to, care for, and suffer with.

It was evening and everyone was utterly exhausted by the time she came out of surgery. My family went up to her room and were amazed that she was sitting up in the chair next to her bed. Her nurse was charting on his computer with his back facing Danielle. While the nurse spoke to everyone and provided a short update, the color slowly drained from her face. My mom kept one eye on Danielle and one on the nurse who was not paying any attention to his patient. Another minute went by and Danielle was now as white as a ghost and barely awake.

"Oh no, look at her! We need to get her to a bed right now. She's going to pass out!" My mom yelled.

If this were a patient of my mom's, she would have jumped into action and would not have been too worried because she's seen this happen before with post-operative patients. Thankfully, this is how Steve reacted. He remained calm and knew what needed to be done. Bill and my mom however, did not. They were both thinking and acting based on fear. Not being in the medical field, Bill had never seen someone pass out and although my mom had, her much stronger mom card trumped her nurse card.

Danielle's nurse turned to look and agreed that something was amiss. Though it seems like it was rather soon to have her sitting up, from what I've witnessed, the present post-operative trend is for patients to get up and move in more normal ways as soon they are able. The nurse was just following orders by having her upright. However, for Danielle, this was clearly too soon. Her blood pressure was only 70 over 34. Normal blood pressure, generally speaking, is 120 over 80.

They got her back into bed rather quickly and called for backup. The doctor on call was alerted about her drop in blood pressure, and for fear of the internal bleeding that could cause a drop like that, they ordered a CT scan of her stomach and a chest x-ray. Luckily, both came back negative and her pressure eventually came back up. She just wasn't ready to join the party yet.

On Friday morning, Steve arrived back at the hospital at 4:00 to make sure Danielle was doing well. He did not want to take any chances and he needed to fulfill an act of contrition from the first night of her first ICU stay back in 2011 when his gut told him that he should have stayed with her. My mom and Bill joined him a few hours later and after realizing that she was doing okay, they both headed home and left Steve to watch over her. It was a fairly uneventful morning until they came to take out her catheter, which made Danielle very excited.

It's normally a smooth and speedy process but without thinking about the major abdominal surgery she had the day prior, Danielle sat back and tried to hoist herself up in the bed. To anyone who has had stomach surgery or a C-Section, you can appreciate the fact that your mind thinks you are capable but your very sore belly does not. She yelped as she popped backward and then popped forward because it was so painful. It actually knocked the breath out of her lungs. It made her panic because she felt the loss of air in her system. It was a double whammy motion that would eventually come back to haunt her.

When this happened, Steve was standing outside of her door, about 10 feet from Danielle's bed, giving her some privacy. As a doctor, he knew Danielle was going to be elated to get the catheter removed. He's seen it done hundreds of times and has done it himself for others. Yet, when he heard her scream in pain, he couldn't understand what could have possibly occurred for that reaction. He thought to himself, "getting a catheter removed is like heaven for everyone so why would she be in pain?" He wondered if Danielle wasn't as pain tolerant as he thought and he incorrectly assumed that she might not be as tough. He quickly realized his guess was incorrect and that Danielle was trying to be *too* tough.

The nurse removing the catheter didn't waste any time letting Danielle know her limitations.

"Danielle you can't do that just yet. Everything is still very tender. I will bring you a makeshift pillow that we put together out of socks that you can use to prop against your torso to act as a buffer. It will help absorb any motion you have in that area."

She abided by the rules for the rest of the day and was visited by our dad who packed his bag and booked a hotel room near the hospital so he could take a turn watching over her.

Before I get into the extremely awkward exchange that our father had with Danielle's Mennonite roommate, I feel compelled to share with you some more backstory on our Dad. As I mentioned earlier in the story, he does things his own way and often he appreciates getting a rise out of us just for fun. But, he would do anything for you and is also extremely loyal – all qualities that he inherited from his own father, my very Italian grandfather, Andrea "Hank" Certo Sr. and his mother, Natalie, the wonderful woman I'm named after.

We called my grandfather "Nonu" which is a take on the Italian word for grandpa, "Nonno." As kids, my cousins and I adored him. He was a rotund man with a bald head and generous spirit. If you showed him your report card, he would reward you with money for working hard. He was quick with a joke and was a very well-known business man in Niagara Falls. He was the type of guy who seemed to know everyone everywhere he went.

He was also not shy when he had a thought he needed to share. At church on Sundays if he thought the priest was taking too long with the Homily, he would yell out to the whole parish "time!" so that the priest could be more cognizant of the minutes ticking by. He had places to go and people to see and he figured Jesus would agree that the priest was taking way too long.

He and Natalie were the proud parents of eight children, Peter (RIP), Cathy, Hank (our dad), Marie, Joe, Kenny, Margaret, and Mark. Nonu also held the honor of being a WWII veteran. More specifically, he was a member of the special group of men who showed exemplary fortitude by storming the beaches of Normandy, France six days after D-Day. A day that happened to also be his birthday, June 12, 1944. Instead of celebrating with a cake and candles, he braved his young life fighting the evil that had taken over Europe.

[Because the world works in mysterious ways, Danielle's daughter May was born three weeks early and came into this world on June 12, 2010, a mere 10 months after our Nonu had passed away.]

His wartime stories were not all distressing, though. After family gatherings, we would sit around the table and snack on post-dessert treats, which included hard nuts you had to crack open, oranges and figs (which were my favorite), and listen to him speak. As a skilled raconteur, we were all wide-eyed as he regaled us with his funny tales. My favorite included a broken heart and a woman on a mission.

As an attractive young GI, my Nonu would have made any girl feel lucky. So, when he received a letter in the mail from a woman he called Lucille Friedel, he thought he had found the woman he was going to marry. I'm not sure why she wrote to him or how she even knew who he was, but she wanted to communicate her appreciation for the boys in uniform and specifically to him. He told his family that he would marry this girl eventually and was excited at the thought of meeting her. What he didn't expect, though, when flipping through the military's *Stars & Stripes* magazine was that his dear Lucille had written letters to GIs all over the country. There was an article in the magazine with a title resembling the following, "Lucille Friedel, Champion Letter Writer." Apparently, she preferred quantity over quality.

Eventually he got over his infatuation with the skillful letter writer and fell in love with my "Nana," Natalie Bator, a beautiful but very Polish woman who worked at Certo Brothers back in the early 1950s. It was a bit of a scandal back then for their love to blossom publicly since she was not even a little Italian. They married anyway and she became the ultimate stay-at-home mom, rearing their brood of eight. She was tough because she had to be and meant business when she spoke. She adopted a lot of the Italian ways of cooking and can knit an afghan with her eyes closed. She's also had her fair share of casino luck. She's won big, over $100K, playing the slots in Atlantic City. Now that she's in her 90s, she's a wonderful great-grandmother and goes by the new moniker, "Big Nana." She and our Nonu bickered back and forth with one another until the day he died in 2009. He passed away peacefully in his sleep. Though he's been gone for over a decade, there is not a day that goes by that his presence isn't felt or that she wishes he were still here. Theirs was a love story for the ages.

Now that you know who and where my father comes from, I hope you enjoy the silent embarrassment that poor Danielle had to endure the day after her first surgery.

When my dad arrived for his visit with her on Friday, she motioned for him to get closer so she could speak to him as privately as she could without her Mennonite roommate overhearing their words.

"Dad, I would appreciate it if you would not befriend my roommate. I'm sure she's very nice but I don't really want to make small talk all throughout the day. I don't mind chit chatting with others but I'm in a lot of pain and I just want to focus on getting home. I know she's had a long road with UC and I overheard her saying she almost died many times from it. I have my own stuff to worry about though right now. Please, please, please just leave her alone."

"Sure D., no problem," my dad quickly replied.

Although her childhood nickname was Bijou (bee-jew), he called her "D" now that she was grown up. Did he listen to his daughter's request, though? Even for 10 minutes?

As he took a seat under the only TV in the room, which was affixed to the wall, halfway between Danielle's bed and the other woman's bed, he couldn't help himself. Danielle could only see him because the curtain between them was pulled. He, however, had the pleasure of seeing them both.

At first, it started with simple pleasantries. Our dad is quite skilled at carrying on a conversation with just about anyone. He's personable and genuinely curious to learn about other people and their story.

"Hi, how are you? I'm Hank Certo."

"Hello there," she said softly.

Then he shifted gears and begin to dig a little further into her background.

"So, I see your Amish?" he implored.

"No, I'm a Mennonite."

"Oh, that's the more liberal sect, huh?"

Danielle put her head in her hands because she knew they were now in for a bumpy conversational ride.

"What? No, that's not the case at all. We are not," the woman argued.

"You drive, don't you? You have electricity, don't you?"

"Absolutely not!"

The woman then became infuriated with his flippant statements and defended her religion as if she was Joan of Arc while our father casually goaded her on for sport.

Their rancorous banter went on for a few more minutes before he gave up and focused back on Danielle who gave him the stink eye.

"Dad! Knock it off! Stop it right now!" Danielle begged.

Couldn't he just have kept his big mouth shut?

Nope, he was not capable of it.

Side note on the poor Mennonite woman – she was also blind and wouldn't be able to change her new appliances on her own like Danielle could. She had to have someone from her church come twice a week and do it for her. Sometimes when you think you have it bad, there is someone else nearby who has an even heavier cross to bear – a fact not lost on Danielle throughout any point in her story.

Our Gram taught us that, often repeating, "If you are sitting around a table with your closest friends, and everyone reveals the cross they are currently bearing, you will quickly grab hold of yours and keep it because others almost always have it much worse."

Danielle stayed positive and held onto those words even when she started to bleed out of nowhere.

Early Saturday morning Danielle felt strong enough to take a lap around the floor. My father had gone home because Bill was due back later in the day. The doctors and residents on call had just reached her floor and were being updated by the nurses before they rounded on their patients when Danielle happened to stroll by the group. She smiled and unknowingly began to bleed from her stomach onto her baby blue hospital gown. At first, she didn't realize it was happening until one of the nurses spotted the insidious red circle forming. She was immediately sent back to her room to lie down. The bleeding was steady and they determined it was coming from her belly button, one of the sites that the surgeon used, via the robot arm, for the surgery. The surgeon was then alerted to the situation but when she arrived to examine Danielle, she was not confident that the bleeding was coming from anything she had done on Thursday. Since it was not gushing out of her, they decided to wait and see and address it in a few hours. She figured they could assess the situation better based on an increase or decrease in the volume of blood they could see seeping through her bandages. The surgeon explained that if ultimately it was something related to the surgery site, they would have to take her back down to the OR and poke around until they found the culprit.

During this time, Mike, the kids, and I were all en route to Rochester to see Danielle and to see our good friends who happened to also live up there. Our plan was to put our kids down for a nap at our friend's home and then visit Danielle for about an hour before heading back to Olean. With the kids then sound asleep, we very carefully snuck away and headed to the hospital. My mother called though to let me know that Danielle had some bleeding earlier in the day and they were watching to see what would come of it. The hair on the back of my neck stood up and I had the sense that something was amiss. For some reason, throughout Danielle's ordeal, there have been times when I felt deep down in my bones that she would be okay. But then there were times when I knew something was brewing and a shoe would inevitably drop. In this moment, I felt the latter with great certainty.

We arrived to her room and saw her pleasantly laying in the first bed with the curtain drawn to separate her from her roommate. She gave us the update on the bleeding and how it wasn't really bothering her too much. She explained to us that the doctors didn't seem concerned but the nurses were, though, because it didn't seem to be letting up. We then met her two male nurses who were both fantastic. One was a tall, thin gentlemen in his mid-thirties who seemed to be a mentor to the younger nurse who was also training to be an EMT. They were both compassionate and caring and it was clear that they made Danielle's bleeding tummy a priority. We chatted with her only briefly before the hemorrhaging became more intense. The bandages that were covering her belly button became blood soaked very fast. It was as if someone let the dam burst and blood began oozing out at a much quicker pace. Sensing things may get tricky, Mike decided to make more space in the room and left to go get our kids. Everyone involved in her care then moved briskly to stop the floodgates. In the process, bloody bandages and cloths were tossed about and Danielle's bare mid-section was put on display for anyone coming into the room to see.

Since her surgeon had gone home for the day, the surgery fellow (a medical student graduate that has passed the resident stage) was called in to reassess her condition. And to our sisterly delight, he was a young Italian guy (Che fortuna Italiana!) with black hair and an extremely chiseled face. He was there right away and took over the unfolding situation. He was also very kind and decided that perhaps Danielle tore something when she popped back the day before with the catheter removal. He believed the bleeding would possibly stop if he tightly stitched up her belly button site. There weren't enough hands around though to apply pressure so while the dreamy fellow gathered up his instruments and supplies, he asked me to put on gloves and jump right in.

Internally, I panicked!

"What! Me? You want me to get involved and be face to face with the bloody mess happening all over Danielle's stomach?"

This can't be happening I thought to myself. Why

wasn't Steve, the actual doctor in the family, still here?

The answer: Steve was in the unmentionables section of Walmart buying women's underwear. While he had been sitting with Danielle discussing her new reality, he had done some research on the best type of underwear for someone in her condition. Because he knew we were coming to check in, he tagged out and went in search of helpful undergarments.

As someone who despises blood in all forms, I had to step outside of myself and firmly press on my sister's belly for a good 10 minutes while we waited for her to be sewn up. She remained calm and collected even though it was a bit of hairy situation. He numbed the area, cleaned it off with Betadine, and then began his stitching using a very sharp and long needle and a fairly thick suture material. In reality it could have been a small sewing needle and very thin thread but to my wide eyes, it was draconian! I didn't have time to ponder the situation very long before our attention was diverted to the Mennonite parade that suddenly formed at the end of Danielle's bed.

As kids who grew up in Western New York, we were always fascinated with the Amish people who lived out in the country nearby. Which is possibly why our father couldn't keep a lid on it. They dressed differently than us and were taught to live off their land almost entirely. They didn't drive cars in favor of using a horse and buggy and most of them did not have electricity like he suggested. They didn't go to our schools but were schooled together as a group, so we never came in contact with them directly. It was common knowledge, though, that their craftsmanship was unlike any other around. They could build anything, bake anything, and grow anything.

From what I understand, there are varying degrees to being a part of the Mennonite faith, which includes the Amish. Although Danielle's roommate dressed like the Amish we knew growing up, they identified with the "Mennonite" label instead, which we partly learned from our father's extremely awkward conversation the day prior. The parade of people were dressed in the same Amish blue-toned garb, marching in one-by-one as the Italian fellow worked to suture Danielle's exposed and bloody stomach. We watched in disbelief as person after person, including a handful of children, trotted by and huddled around the woman in the next bed. Each one gazed at Danielle with startled eyes as they passed. The only thing missing from this hilarious procession was a peddler selling souvenirs and livestock. We were dumb-founded at the timing of it all but had a good laugh afterwards. What are the odds that she'd bleed so profusely from her surgery site that she'd have to be sewn up while eight part-Amish well-wishers casually watched?

Not any I'd bet on.

While she was being worked on, to distract her mind from what was occurring and the embarrassment of being on display for everyone to see, Danielle had me talk about the fantastic shopping trip we were going to take and the amazing night out we'd have once she was healthy.

"Let's focus on the nice glass of Pinot Grigio you can enjoy when this is all over! And while you're drinking it, you'll be wearing your new soft pink sweater from Ann Taylor. And you'll be sitting on the new champagne colored chenille loveseat that you purchased from Home

Goods."

She was an absolute champ throughout it all. She didn't have too much time to stress over what was occurring because it all happened so fast. Once she was stitched back up and her stomach was not being shown to the world, we took a second to reflect on the craziness that we had just witnessed: a bloody mess all over the place, an unexpected Mennonite procession, and me as Florence Nightingale. Someone was looking out for Danielle, though, because as we were going over the situation, she received the fantastic news that a private room had opened up and if she'd like to pay a small fee it could be hers.

"YES! I will happily take it," she exclaimed with glee.

Bill and Steve arrived shortly thereafter and were told that they did not have to wait long before they were able to blow that pop stand. Before they departed, Bill noticed the Mennonite kiddos peeking from around the curtain and staring at Danielle's TV with their mouths agape. So as the father of two small girls, he found a channel with cartoons and switched the station so they could watch as well.

Her new room was positioned in the corner with a private bathroom and felt brighter and more spacious. She had big windows and the sun seemed to shine in more so than her previous room. Once she was settled and felt at ease, I said my goodbyes and let the men take over. Bill stayed the night with her in a chair next to her bed just to be sure that someone was there in case something else new and fun arose (like a bleeding belly button) and Steve eventually headed home.

She seemed to be progressing nicely by Sunday afternoon and was lucky enough to receive a visit from our Aunt Phyllis, my mother's older sister, and our Gram who was 90 at the time. They did not use a GPS app to navigate their way from Niagara Falls to Rochester and made it despite the odds stacked against them finding it. They did not stay too long but wanted to hug Danielle in person and let her know they'd been thinking and praying for her all along the way. It was an uneventful visit (thank God!) but one that succeeded in boosting Danielle's morale.

By Monday she was almost ready to go home. In order to receive her discharge papers, she was required to change and clean her whole ostomy bag appliance from start to finish while a nurse looked on. In preparation for that test, the very nice bearded nurse who helped her when she was bleeding gave her a few pointers. Danielle remembers hearing those pointers with a blushed face of embarrassment. She had been trying to do it on her own while simultaneously trying not to flash the bearded nurse. So, she had strategically placed her gown in all the right spots to keep herself as covered as she could. However, there were a few moments where her bikini bod was on display. He told her it might be easier if she sat while she did it and once she followed those instructions, she agreed it made things a lot easier.

On Tuesday, she was officially ready. She had passed the test and had seen every skin nurse from Rochester to Racine. My mom drove up to bring her home and carefully took it slow the entire way back. Danielle was elated to see her kids, her dog, and her own bed. She was reminded, yet again, how long a week feels when you are away from home and stuck in the hospital.

It was early October and the temperatures were becoming brisker in the morning. There were still many afternoons, though, full of sun and warmth. She took advantage of the nice weather and managed short walks up and down the street to build her stamina. On the first day she could only do about ten minutes before she had to turn back. But each day, things were incrementally better and getting back to work was coming into view for her. The pain needed to fully subside so that she could move through her day without any assistance via her pain medicine. Gratefully, during this time there were no major hurdles and no issues preventing her progress.

When she had to go back up for a follow-up appointment with her surgeon a few weeks later, she stopped at Insomnia Cookies and bought a box of treats for the nurses who took such good care of her. As children of a nurse, we are always aware of the often-thankless job they have, yet, how critical of a career it is. Doctors tend to get most of the credit because they are in charge, but nurses are on the front lines dealing with the not-so-glamorous parts of caring for a patient.

By early November, Danielle was back to work. She had to acclimate herself to the kids she never got to meet but in doing so, she gave them very little information on why she was away. As hormonal teenagers tend to do, they didn't ask a lot of questions. The issues and daily struggles for her during that time were minimal, though, she did constantly live in fear that her ostomy site, the stoma, would leak out stool onto her nice dress clothes and she'd have to run to a bathroom really quickly. She managed that trepidation by being prepared and stashing extra sets of clothes everywhere she could. She also confided in Julie, her teaching assistant, and the school secretary, that she may have a "Code Leaking Stoma" situation in the future and they'd have to take over for a few minutes while she cleaned herself up.

She did have to be mindful of what she ate as well. Things that were thick and starchy, like mashed potatoes and crusty baguettes were helpful because they caused food to move through her more slowly. Drinks like coffee and wine were a little risky because they had a faster trajectory. She tried to moderate her diet as best she could and paid close attention to everything she consumed in relation to her new, super fun accessory.

She also spent a lot of time wishing for Sundays to come. Not because it was a day of supposed rest but because it meant that the start of a new week loomed ahead. On that day she looked for the happiness she would feel because each Sunday there was a reminder that one more week had passed. And that meant one less week she had to live with an external poop holder. One less week that she had to fret over her outfit choices or if her students could see what was under her sweater. With each Sunday, she was one step closer to being done with this never-ending saga.

The weeks eventually passed and time hurled us all forward again to surgery day number two, January 16th, 2017. It was Martin Luther King Jr. Day, and that meant that as a banker, Mike would be off. He stayed home with our children so that I could join my family at the hospital.

But before Danielle could leave her students for the second time, she wanted to share with them a bit more of what she was experiencing. Up until this point, Danielle was private with regard to what her students and most of her coworkers knew about her condition. Given the nature of her issues, it was not a comfortable subject for her to broach with a gaggle of teenagers. Yet, she knew she needed to provide some sort of explanation for her upcoming absence. She felt she owed it to them. She had come to know them well despite having had to skip the beginning of the year due to surgery number one. As a wise educator, she used the tools in her toolbox to "meet" them where they were – with emojis. She created a fabulous PowerPoint presentation that told her story illustrated with the most common symbols. She did not get into particulars but she shared that she had an illness (sad face) and that she had to have surgery (sick face) but that ultimately, she'd be better and would be back to normal soon (happy face). She also shared that she identified with unicorns as a symbol of hope and good luck.

Her affinity for unicorns began before her first surgery. May had snuck a small white and purple unicorn stuffed animal in Danielle's overnight bag so she wouldn't be alone and would have a piece of home with her. And the reason that May so kindly thought to do so is that Danielle joked with my mom and I that when she took her pain medicine at night to try and ease the agony, she was lifted off to "La La" land where magical unicorns danced around her in the clouds. May must have picked up on that notion and decided that Danielle should have a real unicorn with her at the hospital. Kids can be so pure and wonderful at just the right moments.

On the day of the surgery, Danielle rode with Bill and I rode in the backseat with my Mom and Steve.

Thankfully, for a January day, the weather cooperated and we were all able to travel up there with no trouble. Danielle remained composed until the pre-op waiting room when we all came in to say hello and goodbye. She melted into a small puddle of fear, like any normal human, as she waved farewell to us. She did not fall prey to the ugly cry like she had the first time around, but she was weepy still for sure. My mom had to remind her that she had done this once before and would get through it. However, this surgery would be the most complicated of the three.

In very brief, laymen's terms, the highlight of this operation would be the creation of the J-pouch using the end portion of her small intestine. When she was completely healed, this pouch would become her pseudo-new rectum. The pouch would need time to rest and heal so her surgeon carefully and precisely looped the open piece of her small intestine (the piece that came out of her stoma site) so that waste would empty into the bag but nothing would travel down into the new pouch that needed to rest. So, although her stoma site didn't move this time around, the part of her small bowel that would be poking out of her belly would be different. This is an important note to keep in the back of your mind because Danielle would have to deal with the repercussions of this small switch as time wore on.

Going into this surgery, though, her surgeon told her some sobering news.

"Danielle you won't bounce back quite as quickly from this one, although you might want to. You went into the first surgery feeling lousy with a diseased colon and we were able to take that away. With the second procedure, you are going into it feeling much better and afterwards you are going to feel worse due to the invasiveness of the operation."

With that thought lingering in the air as we hopped on the elevator, the four of us headed upstairs to the lobby and waiting area where we sat and stared at the public monitor full of patient ID numbers. She jumped from the pre-op column to the OR column and that's where she resided for a few hours. We passed the time by pacing, reading old magazines thumbed through by hundreds of other families, and eating lunch in the massive cafeteria in the basement.

A hospital cafeteria always provides for excellent people watching if that is something that intrigues you. It serves its purpose to provide a warm meal for anyone in need but it is also the backdrop for some of life's toughest conversations. Families are forced to make difficult decisions over a cup of coffee and a muffin *or* are celebrating a cure, a new baby, or a positive test result. Then you throw in the staff that whiz in and out either between shifts or on their lunch break. To non-healthcare professionals, such as myself, medical practitioners are champions. And the idea that one minute they could be scarfing down a tuna salad sandwich and the next minute they could be performing an emergency tracheotomy is astounding. Which is why I found myself gazing across the tables trying to construct everyone's story for the day. A welcome distraction from the real reason I was actually there.

Our small group of four perused the meal offerings and settled back together to break the tension we felt as the wait wore on. Bill became the champion at our table for making us laugh over a chocolate frosted donut. To know Bill is to know his love of a good Sunday morning donut from our local, family-owned grocery store, Reid's Food Barn. Their donuts are award-winning and for good reason. They are perfect. What's not perfect to Bill, though, is the Bavarian cream filled variety. He much prefers the chocolate glazed angel cream ones. Angel cream is a heavier duty whipped cream and not like the pudding style that is Bavarian cream, Bill's archnemesis. So, on this somber day as we ate our lunch, Bill spied what appeared to be a dream donut in the pastry case of the cafeteria. He analyzed the other donuts that could also be angel cream but decided that the one he chose was "it." He was certain this was going to be the donut of his dreams.

"Steve, this is the one. There is a perfect puff of angel cream on this side of the donut which must mean that's what it is filled with."

Steve questioned Bill's assuredness.

"How can you be sure it is? And let me ask you this. What would happen if you bit into that donut and discovered it was, in fact, Bavarian cream instead?"

Bill paused and delivered his answer in a very serious tone.

"Well, that would be just about the worst thing that could ever happen to me."

This was a funny line that made us all laugh because we knew he meant it but in hindsight, it was telling of Bill's belief that Danielle would be okay, without a doubt. One would think that surgery complications would be equated with a statement like, "that would be the worst thing that could ever happen" but to Bill, he knew she'd be okay and, in this moment, a sneaky Bavarian cream donut was far worse to comprehend. Unfortunately, he was forced to face the unthinkable. His donut choice was incorrect and his taste buds were met with a thick vanilla pudding and not a light and fluffy whipped cream. Despite his earlier declaration, Bill mustered his way through the Bavarian cream and we chuckled at his poor displeasure. He didn't take responsibility for the unlucky choice though.

"Steve, I think this is your fault. Because you questioned my decision, it came true," he teased.

We headed back upstairs and waited another hour or so before Danielle's patient ID number was moved to the post-op column. We were then told to head upstairs to the floor where she would recover while we waited for them to wheel her up. Although the surgery was only about four hours, it seemed that the entire day had been consumed by the time we headed for home. Bill stayed the night and we then took shifts going back up to check on her.

For the first couple of mornings post-op, a flock of med school students would enter her room before the sun was up and use Danielle as a teachable case. They would appear in their starched lab coats and fling open the blinds to wake her up. Then they would analyze her progress in an educational way. Just the way we should all start our morning, with a collection of complete strangers who abruptly end your sleep and want to look at your naked belly.

Sign me up!

With crusty eyes and morning breath, Danielle would have to answer questions and watch as the stu-

NATALIE SMITH

dents collectively observed what she said. As a teacher, she was a good sport about it. However, one arrogant student's actions stick out in her memory from that time period. He came in as if he owned the place and proceeded to rip off her bandage to take a peek at the incision. It caused Danielle immense pain, discomfort, and ultimately anger. In that moment she felt as if she was just a name on a clipboard. He didn't warn her and didn't do it with care or concern – the opposite of what a person needs in that situation. The other students looked horrified. Danielle made sure to alert the nurses and other residents that his behavior was unacceptable.

Going forward, when the flock would arrive, she made them each solemnly swear not to rip off her bandages with such reckless abandon. To paraphrase the incomparable Maya Angelou, "when you know better, you do better." And if this was to be a teachable moment for these students, then this could prove a valuable lesson. Patients are people too.

Despite that minor incident, overall, she was a rock star post-op patient. She moved around well, ate well, and seemed to be heading for discharge a day or two sooner than initially thought.

Until... cue the ominous music...she didn't feel well.

It started out slow and began with a fever (get out your shot glass again)! They came in low, usually around 99 or 100, and didn't last too long. Yet, they existed just long enough to make her feel lousy. She would vacillate between being freezing and sweaty based on the medicine she could take that would help alleviate the rise in her body temperature. When her surgeon came to check

184

on her to see what was going on, because Danielle kept telling the nurses she didn't feel well, she insisted that Danielle was fine.

"You just had major abdominal surgery Danielle. It's all connected to that. The fevers aren't spiking too high so you just need to accept this as part of your recovery and try to rest."

Danielle wanted to believe her doctor but internally felt that there was something wrong. How could she have gone from Stevie Nicks to having fevers so quickly? Wouldn't the fevers have come first if it was truly part of the recovery process?

She somehow managed to get her hands on a thermometer and began tracking her temps on her own; an act she was extremely familiar with having done it many times through the course of her disease.

Thursday and Friday of that week had her still feeling cruddy throughout the day. Yet, her doctor was still toeing the line that she was fine and needed to try and tolerate her current symptoms a bit longer.

At one point during these feverish post-op days, the lead surgical resident working under her doctor came to round on Danielle. When Danielle explained her symptoms, yet again, and shared that she had been tracking her temps, he broke a common decency rule that we as humans abide by, not to mention one that doctors should also subscribe to – if you are going to make assumptions and place judgment on someone, don't do it while they are still in earshot! He listened to what she had to say and then went out into the hall to report back to his team, and Danielle's surgeon, on all of the notes he gathered on all of the patients in that unit. In a condescending tone he explained that he felt she was fine but "She keeps taking her temperature!" He made the assumption that Danielle was a know-it-all patient who was looking for something faulty in her condition.

Thankfully the door was open and she was able to speak up and defend herself.

A lesson she proudly learned from our Nonu and our own dad.

"I can hear you!" she hollered.

How dare he begin to know why she was taking her temperature? He didn't know her. He didn't know her journey. And clearly, he didn't know why it feels validating to see rising numbers on a thermometer when you suddenly feel like a limp dishrag and everyone is saying that you are "fine."

He wasn't contrite in his response and just reiterated the statement, "Well, you are taking your temperature quite a bit."

Though the fevers never really subsided, they didn't get worse so Danielle was able to go home on Saturday.

From the outside looking in, what should have been a joyful occurrence felt uncertain to me. I remember believing that she wasn't ready and something did not feel right. In talking with her and in looking at her, it was pertinently clear that she did not feel good and that her unwell status went beyond the pain and displeasure of someone recovering from surgery.

My mom had the girls so Bill could get her home

and settled in before they came to greet her. She found her way to the couch almost immediately and did not move much for the rest of the day because she was still feeling ill. She didn't have any bounce in her steps and wasn't able to do anything other than take it easy.

Her discharge instructions included an important note – if her fever ever reached 101 degrees or higher, she needed to get to the ER as soon as possible. She had been tracking her temperature closely from the time she had gotten home to ensure she did the right thing. And in doing so, the readings on the thermometer reflected what she already knew. She did not feel better.

On Sunday, she actually began to feel worse. By that afternoon, when they saw the thermometer read 101, they called me and I came to babysit so she could go to our local hospital to be seen. Steve and Bill accompanied her while my mom and I, along with Bill's mother Rhonda, sat at their kitchen table and worried. Their girls were fast asleep while the three of us feared the worst.

"Mom, could her bowel have been obstructed and the fever is a result of stool seeping into her bloodstream?" I questioned.

"I hope it's not sepsis entering the picture again. That was awful for her the first time she got sick," my mom declared.

"Sue, if they can't figure it out, could they go back in and explore the area to determine the cause?" Rhonda wondered.

My mom couldn't have known for sure but admitted that was a possibility.

After being examined by the ER doctor, our hospital did not want to admit her based on her connection to Rochester but they did perform a CT scan of her belly and noticed there was a fluid build-up near her rectum. The GI team on call in Rochester agreed there was something showing on the scan and that she needed to be seen. They gave her the option of coming up right then and there, which was now around 9:00, or waiting until the morning and being admitted through the ER which would get her through the process faster. She opted for plan B so she could sleep in her bed, or try to, one more night.

Steve took her first thing Monday morning so Bill could take care of the girls and get them off to school. The plan went accordingly and they determined, after further testing, that it was, in fact, a fluid build-up based on her newly connected parts draining in one specific spot. Eventually these parts would heal and close up but this was an unfortunate side effect of her recovery process. And because it was "stool-like" fluid, the fevers were a symptom of her body trying to fight it off because it contained her body's waste. Their plan was to go in and insert a drain on Tuesday so she had to spend the night on Monday. Steve stayed with her for moral support and to ease the emotional burden that she'd have once the test was completed.

On Tuesday morning, the radiologist, with the help of x-ray guided technology, inserted a tube the length of two drinking straws and just a bit thicker, directly through her butt cheek (gasp!) that went exactly to the spot where the fluid had been collecting. All in all, he took out 80 ML of fluid. For someone that doesn't understand the metric system (me), that is the equivalent to about a third of a cup. It wasn't an incredible amount but just large enough to be the culprit of her fevers and ill feeling.

The tube coming out of her butt cheek was connected to another tube that was attached to what looked like an IV bag. This contraption was then affixed to her upper thigh via a special strap that loosely looked like a garter and belt. She felt better almost immediately and was able to go home that afternoon. She was not prepared for what she would have to endure for the following 14 days, however.

Prior to this procedure, they did discuss with her the idea that she'd have a drain put in and it would be her new favorite accessory for two whole weeks. They didn't get down and dirty with the size of the drain, how often she'd have to tend to it, and how gosh darn awful it would feel once the Lidocaine wore off. Plus, they failed to remind her that she still had to manage her ostomy bag and keep that site clean in addition to these new responsibilities.

With the new drain now in place doing its job, she needed to clean and flush it out two times a day to keep it sanitary. My mom or Steve came in the mornings to help her with that process and Bill was on duty at night so she didn't have to maneuver through it alone. It was nice and necessary that she have the help but it was not flattering in any way, shape, or form and definitely added to Danielle's slice of humble pie.

As if she needed another reason.

By this point in the game, she'd had to speak to a myriad of strangers about how she poops, watched as a

Mennonite brigade marched past her while she bled from her stomach, and had her rear end flushed out by nurses, and herself, several times. At this rate she was destined for a vacation at a nudist colony by year's end.

Ultimately, she managed the uncomfortable (on multiple levels) cleaning practices okay but did not expect the side order of pain that went along with it. And although in the scheme of one's life, 14 days is incremental; small potatoes one could even argue. However, when you are already living with a bag of poop attached to your stomach, just had your second major surgery in six months, and now have to live with a drain that is literally poking out of your butt cheek, it felt like an eternity to Danielle.

Oh! And the nightly low-grade fevers still existed a few days after the drain was inserted. Eventually they would subside but for a few days, she muddled through her day with an ostomy bag, a protruding butt drain, and daily fever episodes.

She could only sit on one side of her body comfortably and the same went for sleeping, which bound her to the couch so she could lay on one side with support. She tried to endure the pain with the basic pain meds she was given at the hospital but it wasn't cutting it. For the first and last time, because the narcotics laws were changing in New York, she was prescribed Oxycontin. And when that ran out after a few days they readily filled her prescription again. The doctor who performed the drain insertion knew just how awful Danielle was probably feeling and did not hesitate to try and help her. The downside to taking these stronger meds meant that she couldn't drive and it made her feel very loopy. In other words, not only was she frolicking with unicorns in the clouds at night but they would also sit and have breakfast with her each day. She would try to take them only at night when it was bedtime and in the middle of the night when she would invariably be awake. She was typically groggy in the morning but did her best to be there for the girls as they got ready for school. After lunch she would take another pain pill and take a nap before school ended and the girls were due home. Bill then became the rock star who ushered them off to school, worked all day, and then helped Danielle once he came home. Lily and May were also fantastic little helpers who smiled big and didn't focus on the tumultuous time period that encompassed them. Both Bill and Danielle deserve tremendous credit for raising kiddos who adapt well and look on the bright side. Qualities that will serve them extremely well as they get older.

Within the first few days of having the drain, she collected a good amount of fluid, which helped her slowly feel better. By day eight, though, the incessant buttock pain was trumping her ill feeling and it was all she could focus on. She pleaded with her surgeon to have the drain removed sooner but was unsuccessful with her request.

"Danielle, I understand your discomfort but if we remove it too soon and the anastomosis isn't fused together all the way, you'll end up where you started, the fluid will collect and you won't feel well. And then we'll have to insert the drain again and that is not an outcome either of us want for you."

For those of you who don't know what an anastomosis is and would like to use it in your next game of Scrabble, it's the connection that's made when you surgically join channels of the body together (i.e., blood vessels or parts of one's intestine). The more you know!

Danielle hung her head low and put her phone down feeling painfully (no pun intended) defeated. Six more days of this awful existence seemed like cruel and unusual punishment. She tried to dig down deep and get through it the best that she could but it was a tough task. By day 10 she called back.

"Please, please, please. I'm begging you. I can't do this anymore. I can't live in this pain. My mom is a nurse, my step-dad is a doctor. They can help me take it out. I don't need to come up and make an appointment."

She received the following answer from her surgeon. An answer delivered in a curt tone. And here's why: throughout the drain ordeal, her surgeon was not impressed with the idea of inserting it, and she was not impressed with the amount of fluid that was taken out. She believed that Danielle could have managed the fevers and eventually they would have gotten better. So, Danielle's relentless requests were probably just one more task to be addressed by the very busy surgeon.

"Okay. If you want it out, then you need to go to a hospital and have it done by a radiologist because a radiologist put it in. Additionally, it needs to be a sterile environment because we can't risk you developing a secondary infection."

Yippee! Curt or not, she got the signed permission slip.

Because Steve was a beloved physician at our local hospital at that time, he was able to connect with the wonderful radiologist on duty that day and she quickly agreed to make Danielle one happy lady. It didn't take her long to remove the literal thorn in Danielle's backside. Relief swept over her and Danielle's gratitude for that radiologist was (and is) tremendous. Now, finally, she could begin recovering from her surgery without the awful drain distraction.

Essentially, it was onto the next problem.

Remember when I pointed out that the intestine coming out of her stoma site was different this time around? Here's that small piece of intestine's 15 minutes of fame. Because that area had been altered, she began to have major issues creating a clean seal from the stoma to her ostomy bag without the caustic stool seeping outside onto her skin. For some anatomical reason, there was a divot in the area where the site existed and the configuration of the intestine peeking out created trouble for her. Thus, it was extremely difficult to find that perfect seal that would protect her skin from the irritation of having the stool hang out where it shouldn't. Try and try as she might, Danielle was very rarely able to seal it well. And when she did, she would try to hold out as long as she could from having to change and clean the area so that she didn't have to fight through it as much. That was a rare occasion, though, and as the days ticked on by, the skin around the stoma site looked as if it had been through a meat grinder. With the help of her ostomy NP's phone suggestions, she tried every type of cream and potion under the sun to halt the damage but was never really able to alleviate the discomfort.

The end of February was upon her and she was due to go back to school. Despite her frustration and skin pain, the show had to go on and her students needed her.

On the first day back she donned a gorgeous silk skirt and matching cashmere sweater from J.Crew. Sometimes a great outfit sets the tone for how you feel about yourself, or at least for how you *want* to feel about yourself.

She made it through the majority of the day successfully before trouble began to volcanically erupt underneath her sweater. She left her classroom and headed for the ladies' room. The teacher facilities at her school are single units that are directly off of the hallway where the kids pass by. So, all that separated Danielle from everyone else in the building was a single door where she stood, leaking stool from her stoma site. Amazingly, the stool hadn't reached her clothes but she had to strip down naked while she tried to assess the situation and come up with a solution that would last just one more period before school ended. The bell rang and she was still naked and incredibly flummoxed to be in this position. With her heart racing she was able to get a good enough closure on the site to last her until she got home. She had fussed with it, wiggled it just so, and was able to close it just barely in order to keep from it oozing out onto her belly. She pulled up her skirt as the students whizzed by the door and tried to act composed as she headed back to her room. She knew from that day forward she needed to stash clothes once again and have a better plan should this awful situation occur. Once more, she enlisted the help of her friends and co-workers in case she needed to get to a bathroom ASAP. They employed her code words and knew just what to do if she got into trouble. She assured them that the potential covert missions she had to lead would only last until surgery day number three, April 27th.

Once during this time period when we were happily shopping at my family's favorite store, TJ Maxx, I witnessed the horror of her leaking stool in a public place. It was a chilly day and Danielle had on jeans and a fabulous white vest with a gold stripe from the Gap. We had just walked in with the desire to partake in some retail therapy when I noticed a smallish brown stain on her vest. Somehow, she had sprung a leak and needed a quick plan. Regrettably, she didn't bring a change of clothes with her so while she was in the bathroom, we bought her new pair of leggings and she was able to get herself situated so that she could enjoy the rest of our shopping excursion. She had a smile on her face the whole time and truly rolled with it. She was able to clean and salvage her beautiful Gap vest and continue to wear it, no harm, no foul.

If it had been me in that situation, I know I would have been horrified and probably would have cried in the bathroom. Danielle didn't, though. She handled it with aplomb. An enviable quality that she honed as her ordeal unfolded over the years.

She knew what to do if a leak sprung again but her skin was still dreadfully irritated. Like the pebble in the shoe analogy I used earlier, her skin irritation at this point represented a rock. It was hard to focus on anything else because the discomfort was so great. It burned and ached all at the same time, just about every minute of the day because it was constantly being aggravated.

After a month of living with it and the corresponding fear that she'd spring a leak at any point, she knew she needed to find a better solution to make this problem go away. That decision was solidified one Thursday night when she could not get a good seal. She was up all night long trying her darndest to secure her appliance to her skin without fluid leaking out. She glued and unglued (with the medical-grade kind) the pieces together until zero cows came home because all of her attempts were unsuccessful.

She sobbed.

She hung her head.

And then she silently whimpered.

She looked at herself in the bathroom mirror with puffy eyes and a frown on her face and knew that she could not suffer through another night of fighting with her ostomy bag accessories.

If you are wondering what could have been so difficult for her to do, here is a brief explanation of what she was up against. Remember how her attention-hungry intestine came up and out of her stomach just a bit and that's called the stoma? Well, that bit of tissue is pushed through a flange, which is the collar or flat rim that snaps onto the ostomy bag. The flange is affixed to her stomach by something called a wafer, which on one side sticks to the skin, and the other side sticks to the flange. In a perfect system everything fits completely together and there are no holes or cracks.

Unfortunately, Danielle's system was not perfect.

My mom described how the appliance worked and why Danielle struggled, "The wafer goes right on the skin and has the consistency of caramel. Think of the thick caramel that coats apples for candied apples, that's what it feels like. You peel off the back and that goes onto the skin first. The other side connects to the flange which encompasses the stoma. Then, when you need to empty the ostomy bag there's a little lever that releases the stool so you don't have to change all of that every single day. In Danielle's case, her stoma didn't protrude as much after the second surgery so the flange couldn't hold it in place as well and it created a lot of leaking for her."

Geez, is that all?

The morning after she was up all night trying to get a good seal, she was mentally and physically exhausted. Yet, she felt as if she were in crisis mode. She decided to leave work early that Friday and rushed up to Rochester to see the wonderful NP for some answers. Though the NP had no open appointments that day, she stayed true to her sympathetic mission to help her patients and agreed to see Danielle. Anxious, tired, and extremely frustrated at the agony she'd been enduring, my mom had to drive her up because she was too distraught to focus on the road.

Enough was enough.

The NP looked at the site and offered different bandages and other medical glues that could possibly help. She told Danielle that unfortunately she had to bear with it because her next surgery wasn't too far away and there wasn't much else that could improve the condition of her skin.

"If you were going to be living with the ostomy bag for the rest of your life, I would recommend plastic surgery so that the physiological divot on your abdomen that's causing all of this havoc could be flattened out. But for now, I'm running out of options. I'm really sorry. You just have to live like this for a little bit longer until the next surgery."

It was unfortunate news but it was news that she had to accept. There were no alternatives other than putting one foot in front of the other and doing the best she could to get through each day.

Though there were still hard days all throughout March regarding her raw and bloody skin surrounding her stoma site, she had her eyes on the prize. The date of her third and final surgery was officially in view.

She just had one hoop to jump through in order to be cleared for the procedure — a test to make sure there was no longer a leak with her newly connected parts. The test was in early April in Rochester so she and Bill decided to make it a fun night away. They shopped a little and had a fabulous meal at a nice restaurant. Danielle was in a great mood. She could see the finish line ahead of her and it didn't seem too far away.

What she didn't see, though, as she looked ahead to her future, arrived on the morning of the test in the form of a very large tube that needed to be inserted directly into her rectum.

Poor Danielle and her tubes.

She yelped in pain when they shoved a nickel-sized tube in her rear end in order to inject dye into her system. Then they watched the dye as it traveled through her body and kept a close eye out for leaks.

"How does it look?" Danielle asked the radiologist who performed the test.

"I would say it looks okay but you'll have to talk to your surgeon."

Thankfully, they didn't have to wait long for the

official results and were able to go directly to the surgeon's office to see if it was successful. She and Bill arrived still riding a wave of positivity.

The wave immediately crashed down hard as her doctor explained that the test needed to be performed again.

"Just to be completely sure, we need you to repeat the test, Danielle. There is one area that we are looking at and we can't risk being uncertain with any areas."

So, once more Danielle had to endure a fat tube shoved in a place where a fat tube shouldn't be shoved. And once more they headed back to her doctor's office.

"We're really sorry to deliver this news, but it looks as if there is still a spot that needs more time to heal. We cannot move forward as planned with the April 27th date. We need to push it out further by at least six weeks. We will perform this test again as the new date gets closer but our hope is that you'll be ready by then."

Danielle put her head in her hands.

"What? I can't go another six weeks like this."

She was despondent.

How could the world be so cruel?

I'll tell you how:

-    She was hospitalized in the ICU in 2011 with sepsis and then was back in a hospital bed again in January of 2012 from the sulfa reaction.
-    She was back in the hospital in May of 2016 after, through the grace of God, somehow making it through a three-day trip to D.C. as the lead chaperone.

- Then, because the first biologic medicine didn't work, she found herself hospitalized thirty days later.
- Three months after that, in September of 2016, after another failed round of medicinal infusions, she had her large colon removed and was given an ostomy bag and a bloody stomach.
- Then in January of 2017 she had her second surgery with a side of fevers and the additional fun of a tube drilled into her buttock. She was then blessed with constant skin pain and irritation.

And now this.

She had to wait another month and a half for this bad dream to end.

They left the hospital and headed for home. She then did what any red-blooded woman would do when given soul-crushing news. She cried into a pint of decadent fudge ripple ice cream and watched classic sappy movies like *Steel Magnolias* and *Beaches*.

Just kidding!

She got chickens.

Yes, you read that right. Bill built a chicken coop in their bucolic backyard and they bought a six-pack of newly-hatched chicks from Tractor Supply Co. With the aid of a warming lamp, they watched as these new members of their family grew into hens which they quickly named: Rosita, Virginia, Henrietta, Daisy, Wanda, and Morgan.

Prior to Danielle's soul-crushing news, my mom and Steve had toyed with the idea of getting chickens and had even purchased a small hen house. However, given the situation with Danielle, my mom couldn't pull the trigger.

"I couldn't possibly deal with chickens, Steve. Danielle is just too sick," she explained.

Steve completely agreed. Her next statement was questionable, though.

"I know! Let's give it to Danielle."

What a solution, Sue!

It was faulty logic for sure but in the long run, it was the best option for everyone involved.

With Danielle's numerous health challenges, my mom never found the time to execute their poultry plan. But because Danielle was looking for a way to kill time and distract herself from the extra days she was forced to wait, the hen house found a new and welcome home with Danielle and Bill. Lily and May were over-the-moon with their new pets and have been the sole caretakers of their "girls" ever since.

In case you've seen Jennifer Garner's Instagram account and now think that taking care of chickens looks glamorous and desirable, here are a few things you should know:

1. They poop. Everywhere. Danielle and her girls had to designate certain shoes as "chicken shoes" so that they could keep track of which shoes ventured into the danger zone that is their coop. Those particular shoes stay outside at all times and under no circumstances enter their home.

2. They eat bugs. And ticks! +2 points for the chickens.

3. They also like to pick and fling mulch. -2 points for the chickens.

4. They like to wander into neighboring yards but are easily herded back with treats.

5. When laying eggs, they start out strong. But as they age into womanhood, their egg laying abilities diminish. Same girls, same.

[2021 update: Only one of the six original hens remain. The others went to the big chicken coop in the sky. They have however added new gals to the mix so the older broads have a younger cohort to hang around with.]

The moral of the story, though: get yourself some farm animals when the going gets tough. Because in April and May of 2017, their six feathered friends provided a break from the treadmill of sadness that Danielle had been running on for months. And although Lily and May weren't overtly worried about their mom, they were still witnessing and experiencing the process through their own childlike perspective. So, those glorious little feathered friends indirectly helped them too.

CHAPTER 10

As we neared Memorial Day and folks in our neck of the woods were planting their gardens and buying hanging baskets of beautifully colored petunias, Danielle had a small list of things to tackle before she could go under the knife: let her students in on why she would be absent for the rest of the year and undergo the dye test once more.

She decided once again to reach her students on a level they could relate to. This time she went with turquoise and purple unicorn cupcakes, baked and decorated by yours truly. Unicorns were exploding in pop culture at the time and given Danielle's existing connection to the mythical creature, it seemed like a natural fit. Ultimately, it was a fun gesture and it lightened the potentially sad mood of having to say farewell. I made almost 90 cupcakes for her that day and I felt tremendous gratitude that I was able to be a part of her send off. Her students really appreciated being told the truth and the experience was cathartic for Danielle. It allowed her to close off that school year knowing that she wasn't leaving them with unanswered questions.

Telling her students: check.

All that was left was enduring the dye test. For obvious reasons, the stakes were extremely high. Did she have the mental tenacity to handle bad news again if her new parts were still not healed? Would they need to invest in more barnyard animals if she received another crushing blow?

I could hear my phone conversation with Danielle if that came to fruition, "hold on Nat, one of the cows got out again, I need to let you go. Mabel, get back here right now!"

The new tentative surgery date was set for Thursday June 1st and the determining dye test was set for the Tuesday before – a buffer of only two days. My mom drove her up to the appointment and although they were hesitant to get their hopes up, at least Danielle knew what to expect and was prepared for the extremely uncomfortable procedure. She had taken some medicine beforehand in order to fight the agony of having the wide test tube shoved up her rear end for round two.

Once it was over, they were sent to see her surgeon.

On this day, however, they were given the green light.

"You passed the test. The surgery on Thursday is a go!" The surgeon happily explained.

Danielle was filled with jubilation. Trumpets roared in her head. Finally, this nightmare would come to a conclusion. And thankfully, she did not have to wait too long for her new dream to come true.

The smile from Tuesday's good news had not left Danielle's face. When she was wheeled away to the surgical suite the morning of the surgery, she was not sad or scared. She didn't weep or wilt. She was ready to complete the process and no longer wear her excrement on her belly. She was ready to start the new chapter.

I remember that day well because it was my son Sawyer's second birthday. It was a blessing that he was too little to remember the nervousness that was probably written all over my face. I sat this surgery out because my daughter Sadie was in pre-K at the time and I was home with him. I had to rely on Danielle's tried and true trio of supporters: my mom, Steve, and Bill. Luckily this surgery was always going to be the fastest and least invasive. Her surgeon's task this go around was, in simple terms, to remove the ostomy bag and connect her new internal J-pouch to her rectum; essentially making her digestive tract one, long cohesive route from start to finish.

The surgeon came to see the three of them once she was finished and shared more good news. The surgery went well and she did not foresee any complications. They were thrilled and started disseminating the information to the rest of us who were waiting on the sidelines.

From her shaky memory, Danielle remembers one very important moment in the recovery room.

With her eyes closed and her brain somewhat still asleep, she grabbed for her ostomy bag.

"Is it gone? Is it gone? Please tell me it's gone!"

The recovery room nurse smiled and replied.

"Yes, Danielle, it's all gone."

It must have been a buy one, get one free day in the surgery department because the recovery room was extremely busy and she had to wait a bit longer than usual. Because of the prolonged wait time, Danielle kept falling in and out of sleep as the anesthesia was wearing off. The kind recovery room nurse who answered her initially had to keep answering the same question because poor Danielle couldn't remember.

Thankfully, because of Steve's occupation as an anesthesiologist, I used his vast knowledge of sleep-inducing medicines to understand why this phenomenon occurs for patients post-op. He explained the following:

"Ditching the ostomy bag weighed on Danielle's mind pre-surgery and as she was being put under, that was probably the last conscious thought she had. Then, among other medicines, she was given Versed to relax her. Versed is like valium and its effects mimic the sensation one has after drinking a few glasses of wine. It also causes something called retrograde amnesia, which is the inability to recall past memories."

Therefore, the *Groundhog Day* conversation happened a few more times.

"Do I still have it? Is the ostomy bag still here?"

"No honey, it's all gone. You don't have to worry."

Eventually, she was wheeled up to her private room to meet her merry band of well-wishers. My mom, Steve, and Bill were also extremely relieved to know that it was gone and her life could and would resemble normalcy to some degree. It was all over. She had done it.

Friday came and went and Danielle's recovery was excellent. She wasn't eating yet but all of her blood work looked great and so did she. She was heading in the right direction and would need a "shift change" of visitors come Saturday morning. Madison, Noah, and I raised our hands and planned on visiting her for the afternoon.

There was still a slight spring chill in the air when I

got ready for the day. I had just purchased some new summer clothes and was dying to get use out of them. Visiting Danielle, who was doing better than expected, seemed like a great reason to get "dressed-up." As a mom of a two-year-old and a four-year-old, there were not many occasions that I could wear stylish clothing and not get them dirty at the hands of a child. So, on that morning I was feeling happy for Danielle but also happy that I could wear my new flip flops and navy shorts in honor of her appreciation for fashion.

The warm sun was shining bright by the time we arrived and my optimism for Danielle and this stay was still going strong. Because until that point, no one had uttered the word fever, setback, complication or tube. *And* it was post-op day number three!

When we entered the room, Danielle greeted us with a big, toothy, grin. She was in a great mood and seemed up for small talk. She brought us up to speed on her progress and said that she needed to burp.

Or fart.

In other words, she explained, "I need to prove that my digestion system works and flatulence would be a good sign things are moving along the way they are supposed to."

On post-op days one and two she wasn't too hungry. But, on this day, she had eaten breakfast after she woke up. It was a small meal that consisted of eggs and coffee but it was a solid first step. However, she noted that once we arrived, she had "just a little bit of heartburn" going on which was an abnormal occurrence for her. She had mentioned it to my mom and Steve and I didn't know it at the time, but they were alarmed. To them, her heart-burn meant that the digestive process was moving in the wrong direction. Instead of the food heading down with gravity it was backtracking and moving the opposite way because it couldn't go its intended route.

After 30 minutes had gone by, she became a little sleepy so I decided it was probably time for us to head out. I teased her as we said our goodbyes.

"Although I am extremely grateful for the break in child rearing, I suppose we can get out of your way so you can rest. It's not like you need it since you're doing so well!"

"Okay that sounds good. Do you think you could stop at the gift shop and pick up some Tums? They won't bring me some and I can't shake this heartburn."

As an eager little sister who wanted to help, I was happy to oblige and made my way there. Thankfully, the shop was out of them because I was not aware that she shouldn't have taken them at all.

As I was leaving the shop my mom called.

"Hi mom. I just stopped to snag her some Tums but they are all out."

"Nat, is she okay? I just talked to her and she didn't sound good. She said her stomach feels off. And please don't get her Tums. That sounds like a sign that things in her belly are backing up and not moving down like they should."

"Well, I forgot the bag of *People* magazines I brought for her in Madison's car so I was going to run them back up and hang them on her door so I wouldn't wake her. I can peek in and see how she is?"

"Yes, please do and call me right back."

The above statement can be decoded as such: "if you don't call me back ASAP, I will call you in five-minute increments until you answer." Something she would surely do if I didn't pick up my phone.

Madison and Noah drove the car from the parking garage to the front of the hospital while I made the trek back up to her room on the seventh floor. She wasn't asleep when I got there but looked as if she had been hit by a tsunami of nausea.

"Here are your magazines. I was going to leave them on the door so I didn't disturb you but Mom wanted me to check on you. Are you doing okay? Has something changed since we left?"

As the words came out of my mouth, I could very clearly see that she had taken a bad turn in the short time we had been gone. Her color looked worse, her toothy grin was gone and she seemed extremely uncomfortable.

"I feel really sick to my stomach all of a sudden. Like I want to throw up."

"I'm going to get a nurse," I said abruptly.

Each patient room in her unit was positioned like the rays of the sun with the main nurse's station in the center so it didn't take me long to find her nurse.

"Danielle, can you tell me what's going on?" The nurse inquired.

"I was feeling great until lunch time. I've had heartburn and now I feel really sick to my stomach. I feel like I want to vomit."

The alarm bell that went off inside the nurse's head was obvious. Given that Danielle had surgery just two days ago made the idea of her throwing up not a viable option. She couldn't risk ripping open her incision and possibly doing internal damage to her newly connected parts.

Things moved fairly quickly once we all realized that something had surely gone awry.

The PA on call arrived almost immediately and asked Danielle similar questions.

He surmised that everything she had consumed had become stuck in her stomach and was looking for a way out. It's called an "ileus," which means a lack of movement. After the latest surgery, her new parts needed time to "wake up" and start working on their own. Unfortunately for her, they were still asleep. He told her she could try to wait it out a little bit longer or have the contents of her belly sucked out through a nasogastric (NG) tube. He explained that he would insert a tube up her nose, down the back of throat, through the esophagus, and that it would be attached to suction so they could manually remove the items that were not being digested properly.

"I can do it right here in your room and it would probably be in for three to five days depending on how soon your system begins functioning properly again. It's different for every person but it should happen within that window of time."

Panic washed over her.

"Does it hurt? What will it be like for me after you put it in?"

"Well, it won't be comfortable but that won't last too long once I'm done."

Danielle was worried about the pain and discomfort the NG tube would afford. Given all of the horrible procedures she'd had to endure up to this point, who could blame her? Previously she had 19 bags of warm water thrust into her extremely diseased colon, a tube drilled into her butt cheek, and now they wanted to shove one up her nose and down into her stomach.

To provide more insight on the delight of being given an NG tube, when Steve was in medical school in the 1980s, part of his training was to be "blessed" with an NG insertion by a fellow student. And he had to do the same to his partner in return. I don't believe this practice is still customary but its roots were logical. Because it's an uncomfortable procedure from beginning to end, the professors believed that new doctors would recommend it only when absolutely necessary if they knew what the discomfort felt like firsthand. You don't know what you don't know but if you know for sure that having a tube shoved up your nose and down your throat is torturous, you'll know not to put others through it unless it's to their direct benefit.

Because I knew that Danielle was terrified and that it would be cruel to leave her in this moment, I quickly decided to stay put. I called Madison and Noah and told them I would find another way home and would have to skip the Target run that we had planned on. I knew that Shayne and Victoria happened to also be in the area for a high school baseball game and they could potentially get me home. Or in the worst-case scenario, I could always spend the night in a hotel.

I then had to call my mom back. A call I was not looking forward to placing because I knew she'd be worried.

"Okay, here's the update. They are afraid she'll throw up so they've decided to move forward with an NG tube. Danielle is petrified by it but she feels so lousy so I think that's the plan. She wants to lobby for pain meds beforehand because she's afraid it's going to be really painful."

My mom took the news as well as she could and her nursing background helped. She'd seen many NG intubations in her day but as a mom was not comforted to know that Danielle had a blockage. She knew how uncomfortable it was and how much her patients disliked having them. She mentioned that sometimes patients' arms have to be strapped down to the bed because they want to pull the tube out so badly.

"Yikes," I thought to myself.

Danielle was in for some more hospital fun once this tube was inserted. I looked back to check on her and I could see the fear written all over her face. Anxiety washed over her as she became rigid and scared. She then advocated for herself and asked if she could be given medicine to help make the procedure more comfortable.

"Please?" she asked the PA.

Although it's not a common practice to give patients pain meds prior to putting in an NG tube, because it is fairly quick to administer, they made an exception for the very apprehensive Danielle. They administered the meds and within minutes had the right tools in place. They let me stay in the room for moral support, which allowed me to once again be Danielle's bedside cheer-leader while she underwent an unexpected procedure. She gripped my hand tightly as the PA began to insert the tube up her right nostril. She winced in pain so I began our customary distraction technique.

"What kind of swanky sandals will you buy from J.Crew when you get better? I think you should treat your-self to a sundress as well. And while you're at it, maybe some new summer jewelry? Did you get all of the spring flowers you wanted? I bet we could convince mom to take us to the greenhouse once you're better. Remember that time you had a bleeding stomach and had a parade of folks walk by as it happened? That was much worse than this!"

I prattled on and on about shopping while the PA continually pushed the tube further into her body. She did not tolerate it very well and was pretty miserable, understandably so, the whole time. My heart sank for her even though I was projecting an upbeat attitude. I desperately wanted to twitch my nose and have this mo-ment disappear and be replaced by a much happier one. It felt that she always drew the short straw of post-surgery complications. If it could happen, Danielle would have to experience it.

It was over in a matter of minutes and then we watched as green sewage-like sludge began filling a can-ister attached to the wall. The suction was working and immediately Danielle's nausea waned. Her temperament improved as well because the pain meds began doing their job. She quickly became more relaxed. I stayed for a bit longer to make sure she was well enough to be left alone and then I hitched a ride back home with Shayne, the most perfect chauffeur for that moment. She was calm, kept things light, and was very reassuring about Danielle's progress. As I mentioned before, Shayne almost always sees the glass half full and has a beautiful smile even in times of adversity.

Although I knew Danielle was going to be okay, I realized how fast my heart was beating as we drove home. I slowly chewed on the PB & J sandwich that I had packed in my purse for lunch and replayed the afternoon in my head. NG tubes are fairly common and usually helpful, but having a front row seat to Danielle's experience with it, was still a bit hectic and scary. I truly believed this addition to her care would get her over the hump and hopefully headed in the right direction.

It just had to.

Going backwards, in any form, would just be cruel.

Luckily, Danielle wasn't left alone for long. Steve and Lily were in Buffalo watching a traveling performance of *Wicked* when Danielle was adding to her prize-winning tube collection. When the play ended and Steve saw his messages, he left Lily in the care of Erica, Bill's older sister who lives in Buffalo, and headed for Rochester. He stayed the night with her and in the morning was relieved by my father who tagged in. She was doing as well as she could without being able to eat or drink anything. They were giving her sustenance via her IV but it did not satiate her need for a drink. She begged the nurses for some ice chips and eventually they gave in and allowed her that glorious treat. As Sunday wore on, the volume of fluid being sucked out of her stomach became less and less and by Monday, they decided the tube could come out.

She was elated on one hand but also had a terrible sore throat from the tube irritation. They eased her back into eating again and we all crossed our fingers that her new system would be ready this time around. Hours passed by and then it happened...

She tooted.

Yippee!

With the release of air, the doctors knew that physiologically things were happening as they should. Her smile returned with the hope that she could eventually leave her home away from home on the seventh floor.

After two good days with no proverbial hiccups, she was discharged. Her instructions were to stick around her house for two weeks while she adjusted to what her new bathroom routine would look and feel like. She needed to understand how much control she had when the urge came on and also to know what she could and couldn't eat to maintain that control. She listened to her surgeon and didn't leave her street for at least 10 days post-op. She learned when the urge did come, she was able to hold it long enough to get herself to a bathroom. She couldn't wait a minute more. It was instant and it happened often. For the first few days she was in the bathroom an average of 20 times. She never had an accident but was once again back on the commode for the majority of her day. She added more binding foods to her diet (e.g., mashed potatoes, bread, rice) and the number slowly went from 20 times down to 15 and then down to 12 and then settled in right around 10. So, although she was going half as much, she was still pooping, *and* wiping, 10 times a day.

And lest you forget, she had just undergone major surgery!

Although I've been writing about her rear end for over a year, it still didn't immediately occur to me when she was reliving this time period, that her rear end would be as raw and rough as sandpaper from going so frequently. Thus, she dove back into her treasure trove of creams and salves to help her angry, inflamed skin.

My mom helped her acquire a portable, plastic toilet fountain (like a bidet) that she put directly into her regular toilet to help soak her very disturbed hind end. It definitely gave her temporary relief at the end of the day but it was only temporary. As she grew to navigate her diet even more, she realized that dairy products, greasy foods, alcohol, and chocolate, just to name a few, caused her to go more often and wreaked havoc overall. She also noticed that raw veggies made things more uncomfortable and to this day, she stays away from them. And anything with skin on it can be challenging – baked potatoes, apples, etc. She has a shorter digestive tract, thus, the food she consumes has a shorter transit time which doesn't allow the food to be broken down as well. The fear for her will always be a potential bowel obstruction.

Ten days or so into her new life, despite the issues I just described, she was feeling more like herself. She had more pep in her step and decided it was time to brave the real world. She decided on Saturday morning that she would venture out to the grocery store, which is only a block from her house. I happened to be exiting the store when she and Bill were arriving. Although she felt well inside, I thought she looked horrible. And I don't say that lightly. She didn't look sick necessarily but she didn't look like my sister. Her skin lacked radiance and color. And the most startling factor was her weight. She was very, very thin. She wasn't skeletal per say but she was by no means at a healthy weight. She smiled at me and her mouth and teeth seemed so large compared to the rest of her shrinking face. The NG tube, her new, careful diet, and small nightly fevers (yup, they were still clinging on) had all caused her to shed pounds over a period of a few weeks. In reflecting on that time and that meeting at the grocery store, Danielle remembers feeling excited at joining society again. I remember feeling scared for her well-being.

All she needed, though, was some sun on her face and some more calories added to her meals. She worked on both as the days passed and she proceeded well into weeks three and four post-op. By the end of week four she and Bill headed for the Finger Lakes and an outdoor Tom Petty concert. They purchased the tickets when her surgery was supposed to have been in April figuring that by July, when the concert was scheduled, she'd for sure be up and running like normal. They didn't account for the altered timeline but decided to still go anyway. In hindsight it seems like it was too soon, right? They were trying to collect happy memories, though, since so many had been missed thanks to her disease.

Going into the show she had a small fever and knew she wasn't firing on all cylinders. She wanted to make the best of it and brought some medicine to help. She was able to somewhat enjoy the rockin' good time that was a Tom Petty Show (may he rest in peace) and decided that she would keep trudging forward with her summer despite not being 100% better just yet.

At the start of week five she and Bill took the girls

to the picturesque Robert Treman State Park near Ithaca, New York. Again, it was probably too soon but she was a bit naïve and didn't fully grasp her limitations at that time. They brought lunch with them and decided to embark on a five-mile hike – it was two and a half miles out and two and a half miles back. There was a bathroom near the picnic site but at the time of their departure, she didn't have to go. So, onward they went.

Danielle didn't enjoy the scenic hike at all, though, because not long after they set off on their journey, she had the urge to go but nowhere to relieve herself. She resorted back to clenching her fists tightly the entire way and trying to do her best to put one hiking boot in front of another. She knew she had to push herself along but it was in no way pleasurable or relaxing, which is what the goal had been. She was too preoccupied trying not to poop her pants in front of her family.

She realized after that instance that her body would need to be relieved usually within an hour or two of eating. And although she could technically hold it for a little while, by doing so, it would make her feel extremely unpleasant.

[Since that summer day back in 2017, she and Bill and the girls have been back to Robert Treman State Park to do the very same trail. The second time around she was able to fully immerse herself in the beauty the park has to offer. She was amazed that she had even attempted such a feat so soon after all that she had endured. You can't fault a girl with a "new" colon for trying.]

A week after the failed hike, Danielle and her family headed down to Florida for a visit to the most magical place on earth, Walt Disney World, with a side stop at

Clearwater Beach. Again, like the Tom Petty concert, this trip was planned when her surgery was set for April. They decided to still go and stick to their original plan for the girls. Lily and May had also seen many fun activities canceled and rescheduled based on Danielle's health so they packed their bags and hoped for the best that Mickey Mouse could offer.

The first leg of the trip was spent in Orlando. To say that it was hot and sticky is an understatement. If any of you have been fortunate enough to withstand a Florida summer, you know how there are certain cracks and crevices on your body that can sweat like nobody's business when faced with the formidable Florida humidity. Spend just 15 minutes out in the sun, specifically on amusement park pavement, while you are in line for a ride, and you'll be wishing for snow. She was a trooper and had to maneuver going to the bathroom (a lot) while a guest at the park. It was so steamy in the smelly restrooms that when she put down the thin, commercial-grade toilet paper shield on the toilet, it always stuck to her rear end because she was so sweaty. Unlike most people who purposely try not to use a public bathroom in an amusement park, Danielle didn't have that luxury and was forced to use most of them during the four days they spent in Orlando. This was true partly because she was off of her normal routine, but also because she was eating all of her meals at restaurants. Oh, and because she was treating herself to a vacation cocktail in the evenings. When in Roma!

She also had to contend with nightly fevers.

Still.

Despite her adverse vacation environment, she remained positive. Bill got his beloved Pineapple Whip ice cream treat, the girls swam with dolphins at Discovery Cove, and Danielle was grateful to just be there with her people. She saw the good in where they were, figuratively and literally, even though she was not always comfortable. The second half of their trip was more redeeming. They parked themselves on the beach and had a nice, relaxing stay with a lot less public restroom time. She began to believe that life could, and would, eventually return to some semblance of normalcy.

While she was relaxing down in Florida, we were hard at work at home preparing for a huge surprise birthday party for her. She was only turning 39 that year but it seemed like the right time to celebrate her life and all that she was forced to undergo. We booked a venue, sent out invitations, planned the menu, and secretly spoke about how much fun we hoped she'd have. We chose a Luau theme and decided not to tell Bill either. We figured that because he had to carry a heavy load throughout her ordeal it would be a bonus to surprise him as well.

On the day of her party, I could barely eat and I hadn't slept a wink the night before. The butterflies in my stomach multiplied as the day progressed. I could not wait to see her face when she realized what had been done behind her back. The ruse we concocted was that our mom "offered" to watch the kids for all of us (Bill, Danielle, and Mike and I) to go out on the town so we could partake in some adult pre-birthday festivities. The plan was for me to drive and for Mike to sit in the front seat so that when we were getting close to the Country Club where the party was being held, Mike could text our family to say that the guests should all head out to the parking lot so they could greet her en masse. Danielle switched things up on us, though, and decided to sit in the front with me, leaving poor Mike in the back trying to text everyone without being suspicious.

As we headed through town, Mike "suddenly" realized he had forgotten his wallet.

"Oh no. I don't have my wallet with me. I must have left it at the Country Club last night while we were there for dinner. Can we make a quick pitstop to get it before we head to the restaurant?"

Bill's ears perked up and he began to realize what we were up to.

"Geez, Mike. I guess so. I hope we aren't late for our reservation," I said in my best annoyed voice.

Danielle was still delightfully unaware and kept chatting away.

"Our apple trees have exploded this year. I cannot believe the crop. Our blueberries bushes were disappointing, though..."

She kept right on talking as we got closer to our destination. Occasionally I'd toss in an "uh huh" or a "you don't say?" The whole time, however, I was trying not to smirk or simply bust open with excitement.

The Country Club sits on top of a hill and has gorgeous vistas of the Enchanted Mountains that surround the valley we live in. On that picture-perfect night, the view was spectacular. To reach the top of the hill you have to ride along an old red brick road that ends just as the Club enters your view on the right. We were almost to the top and she was still talking about vegetables.

"Did you plant any tomatoes this year, Nat?"

Internally, I was screaming! "Danielle, at this moment I don't want to talk about horticulture! I can only focus on the fact that for a month I have only thought about the moment that's going to occur in three... two... one!"

As we got to the top, Mike and I looked at each other with wry smiles and then turned to look at her. In unison we yelled, "SURPRISE" just as the partygoers yelled it as well.

She lost her breath for a split second and then immediately smiled as she saw some of the most important people to her: my mom's family, my father and Shayne and their kids, Alexis and her other colleagues and friends from work, close friends that are here in town, and her darling girls who were thrilled to be in on the big reveal. When she got out of the car and hugged my mom and dad (who were also teary-eyed) and then one of her 90-year-old grandmothers, the tears began to fall for her.

She had done it. She had made it to colon reconstructive surgery graduation day. Say that three times fast!

A triumphant sensation came over her. She had crossed the finish line and this was her victory lap. She embraced the emotions that were swirling around her as she took it all in. People who loved her had gotten together in one place, with good food, margaritas, and an elegant, rose-adorned cake. They were all there to raise a glass in her honor and in recognition of everything she had withstood to get to that exact point in time. And that was a swell reason to celebrate.

[Not to be outdone, for her 40th birthday, Bill also

planned a surprise. He presented her with two tickets to Nashville, Music City, and a few days of honky-tonking fun for just the two of them!]

CHAPTER 11

Her surprise party was a nice segue into how her life moved forward into the autumn of 2017. Things began to resemble what she would call normal. May started second grade and Lily was going into fourth. She also went back to work in September, without interruption, and began planning for a large home addition; so large in fact, that the contractor called it a "rebuild." They tore down quite a few walls and existing structures so it was as if they were starting from scratch. The construction company broke ground in November and were there for seven months adding 700 square feet to their current layout.

Within the added square feet Danielle was able to have her dream kitchen with speckled marble countertops and a brand-new gas stove with a wall-mounted pot filler.

And not one, not two, but three ovens!

Amazingly, she gets a lot of use out of all three. She can roast a chicken, bake a scratch-crust apple pie, and broil rosemary red potatoes all at the exact same time. Because all three recipes require different cooking temperatures, she is able to cook them and serve them all at once without having to reheat any item when it's time to eat which is a perennial problem for home chefs.

She was also given a desk and wine rack combo

near her new, expansive kitchen as well as a gorgeous master bathroom, a new master bedroom full of windows and soft carpeting, and a tranquil covered patio – all spaces that make her heart happy. Overall, it was a massive undertaking but to Danielle, it was worth every minute and every dollar they spent making it happen.

In the end, after creating their ultimate spa-like master bathroom complete with a stunning walk-in shower and private commode, Bill decided that this peaceful space should just be for Danielle. He relinquished his rights to sully this area and told her as much.

"Danielle, you deserve to have this space just for you. I can use the kids' bathroom. Then I won't worry that I'll make it dirty."

He knew that she still had to be in the bathroom many more times than the three of them combined and graciously recognized that.

Bill, you deserve a cookie too.

Aside from the mess and chaos that ensues when you tackle a major renovation, Danielle was thriving. She had no bowel issues, had no accidents, and taught herself how to go to the bathroom at work without any trouble. She continued to make tweaks to her diet and was able to eat well, generally speaking. When she saw her surgeon for follow-up appointments, she was given good reports. At the final checkup in late fall of 2017, she was *even* given good news.

"Everything looks great Danielle so we don't need to see you again until next summer."

Danielle was ecstatic in her response.

"That's really great to hear! Thank you for everything you have done for me."

Danielle was grateful for her progress thus far and enjoyed the holidays that much more. In December of the prior year, she was able to appreciate Christmas but was always thinking about the second surgery that was right around the corner. This year, she was able to fully immerse herself in the Christmas cheer. It was a breath of fresh air and the icing on her sugar cookie.

As they rang in 2018, she and Bill were anxious to get their addition finished. Progress was being made but it was still a slow process. They could see the end in sight, though, and it helped make the cold days of winter seem less bleak.

What they didn't see was another surgery looming.

On Friday, January 12, 2018, Danielle felt a twinge in her belly. Maybe even a light stomach cramp. It didn't feel awful and it didn't stop her in her tracks. She just happened to notice the sensation after she had gotten home from work that day. Having learned her lesson so many times before, she didn't dismiss its appearance. She noted what she felt, a mild discomfort above her stoma site, and decided to sleep on it. By morning, she felt okay. It wasn't worse and she didn't feel anything other than this twinge. She had breakfast and coffee and began her day as usual. It didn't go away, though, as the hours passed. By dinnertime, she couldn't eat. She and Bill made the decision around 10:00 that evening to call our mom and admit that something was wrong.

"Mom, I don't feel well. I have a pain in my stomach

and I can't seem to eat anything."

Ten o'clock at night is late to call our mother so the alarm bells must have been ringing so loudly for her when she picked up the phone. Yet, she was calm as she spoke.

"Okay. Well if you think you can make it, why don't you get some rest tonight and we can come up with a plan in the morning if it's worse. It could be the stomach flu? It's that time of year and it is going around."

Though she was nervous, her tone was not emotional. She stepped up to the plate as a mom and chief supporter and assured Danielle and Bill that everything would be okay.

Danielle did her best in her own bed to weather the storm of not feeling well but had to move to the couch in the living room; back to her old stomping grounds of illness. She couldn't stand up straight at that point because the pain was too great and when she walked, she almost had a limp. The pain intensity increased but its origin stayed in one spot, over her ostomy bag site. Dawn eventually arrived and she picked up the phone once more.

"It's worse. I was up all night long and now I can't stand upright."

"Okay. Pack your overnight bag just in case. We're going to the ER now," my mom said in a rushed tone.

That's when my mom called me. She didn't want to call me the night before because it was late and because she hoped this mysterious stomach pain would just as mysteriously go away. It hadn't and now she knew she needed to loop me in, just like old times.

The panic in her voice was immediately evident. There was no calmness or cool way about the news she delivered to me. She was scared.

"Nat, we have to take Danielle to the ER now. She's got a pain in her stomach and it sounds like a bowel obstruction."

"What?" I was dumbfounded.

I had no idea that she wasn't feeling well. The same feeling that I had experienced so many times before when things were deteriorating for Danielle immediately found its way back to my own stomach.

"When I spoke to her on Friday morning, she was fine," I protested.

I needed more clarification on what a bowel obstruction meant exactly because although it had been discussed before, I wasn't entirely sure that I really understood the severity of what it could mean.

"It's brought on by a blockage in her digestive tract, and possibly in her new J-pouch, and it causes it to perforate, or rupture. If stool seeps out then sepsis could set in again."

"What would have caused it to be blocked?" I wondered.

"Either adhesions formed, like scar tissue, and they are preventing food from getting through or it's as if there is a kink in a hose. Pressure then builds up and the intestine can balloon out. That then causes it to break open."

Oh, is that all?

Although I love my sister dearly and still needed

her around, part of me wanted to wring her disaster-prone neck. Not because it was her fault in any way, but because I couldn't imagine her having to bear the horrors or what this could mean. And also, because she has such bad luck and I just assumed that we would go directly to the worst-case scenario.

"Okay, I'll come with you to the ER," I said.

My mom picked me up and we headed to the hospital in silence under the gray skies of that January day. It was hard not to let our minds go to a dark place. It was an easy habit to slip back into. We arrived and she was already in an ER bay with Bill by her side. She had been given some pain meds and she said she felt more relaxed and comfortable for the first time in two days. She was able to carry on a conversation fine and seemed to be handling things really well despite the circumstances.

Their plan of action was to get the GI doctor on call to review a CT scan of her belly to determine if there was an obstruction and then they would proceed from there. We all expected that to be the case and were shocked when upon review, he didn't see such an occlusion.

"What could it be then?" we all wondered.

"Her vital signs look good so we really aren't sure. We are going to call Rochester and see what they would like to do given her history."

From this hospital experience, I learned that one surgeon does not like to touch the work of another comrade if they don't have to. So, it was decided that she would be shipped up to Rochester via an ambulance and the team up there could take over. It wasn't an emergency situation but by transporting her in that way, it was presumed that she would be seen and attended to faster. However, it was still a very slow process. She laid there on a stretcher in Rochester's ER department for 2-3 very long hours before they took her back to an ER room. She was parked near the ambulance bay and as she and Bill sat there, they watched a myriad of emergency cases arrive that were worthy of a reality TV show. The cast of characters that were brought in kept their attention and allowed Danielle a temporary distraction. Some were grave situations, some were alcohol-related, and some cases were just downright absurd.

As her wait time kept being extended, so did the immense pain. When they came to check on her, this is how she described it.

"Imagine a hot poker being inserted into your belly and then someone twists it around. That's what it feels like constantly."

Have you ever seen the movie *The Green Mile*? It's a fantastic adaptation of the fictional Stephen King book with Tom Hanks playing the lead. In the movie there is a magical man, played by the wonderful actor Michael Clarke Duncan (may he also rest in peace), who is able to suck out the bad health of those around him. In the ER bay, while her stomach felt as though it was on fire, she thought of that movie and prayed that something miraculous would happen and she would be cured of whatever unexplainable issue was ailing her.

Tom Hanks did not make a cameo, though, and she was stuck feeling terrible.

The nurses tried their best to keep her comfortable and eventually were able to get her up to a room. They ran more tests, took more images of her belly, and ultimately settled on this diagnosis: a stomach virus.

"The stomach flu? Really? Okay. I guess that's what I thought it could be initially." Danielle admitted.

She was relieved to hear the news but was somewhat skeptical that what she was feeling could be a stomach virus. Someone from her surgeon's office explained that sometimes they can settle in various parts of the abdomen and since her blood work and images looked okay that it made sense to them.

She was able to go home later that day, a Monday afternoon, and decided to take the whole week off just to be safe. She figured she needed time to rest and if it was a virus, she didn't want to pass it on. Her house was still in full construction mode so it was a bit tough to get the true rest she needed so at times she would go down to her in-laws so she could garner some peace and quiet. Tuesday and Wednesday came and went and by Thursday, she was not even one iota better. She was walking as if she was elderly and constantly had her hand on her belly for support. She knew what the surgeon had told her but she also knew that the best and wisest move for her was always to trust her gut. Even if it was malfunctioning at the moment. She started to believe something else was happening and stopped believing in the stomach virus theory.

On Friday morning, the pain was intolerable. This was not a virus. She decided to call her beloved PCP to see if maybe he could help her. She needed her "plan" and she needed it quickly because she could no longer toe the line that whatever was occurring would go away on its own. On Fridays his office closes at noon and when she asked for an appointment, the nurse said that they were actually overbooked already.

"Please, please can I be seen? I've been to the ER here in town and also spent a night in Rochester and it's only getting worse. They told me they thought it was a virus but I can't stand up because the pain is too great. I can't go another day like this and I'm not sure what else to do."

She was able to channel all of the angst that existed around her from bouncing back and forth between the various doctors that had spoken to her over the past week. She shared all of it with this stranger and communicated how badly she needed some answers.

Thankfully, it worked.

Danielle's desperation was strong enough that the kind, guardian angel of a nurse on the other end of the phone, relayed the message to the doctor who responded with, "Get her in here right away." He had her get more blood work drawn before she came in and was startled with the results.

"Danielle your pancreas enzymes are off. Something is definitely going on. It could be your gallbladder but you need to get to a hospital soon to prevent it from getting worse."

Why was the PCP concerned about her pancreas enzymes? He was troubled with the thought that she could have pancreatitis (inflammation of the pancreas), of which the implications and effects are scary. In medical school, most students are taught the following axiom, "Don't f$%k with the pancreas." It's a repeated statement because the pancreas plays an essential role in our digestion by converting the food we eat into fuel. And it also helps to regulate our blood sugar.

Pop quiz in case you ever make it to the Jeopardy stage, can you live without a pancreas?

"What is, yes, you can Alex?"

[Sadly, while writing this book, Alex Trebek, longtime Jeopardy host, lost his hard-fought battle with (the tragically ironic) pancreatic cancer. May he rest in peace in game show heaven. I decided to keep it written the way it was before he passed despite a new host taking on the job.]

Surprisingly, you *can* live without it and in my research, I learned you can live without quite a few internal organs including, your spleen, gallbladder, appendix, colon (you now know about that!), uterus, and ovaries.

With pancreatitis, though, it happens when our own digestive enzymes start attacking the pancreas itself. It's serious and can lead to major and very scary complications. It can be treated but you have to catch it right away. One of the causes can be abdominal surgery and some of the signs and symptoms include: radiating pain, fever, nausea, and stomach tenderness. Thus, it was not a far leap to think that this is what she actually had.

She took this information and called Bill and my mom. And when my mom called me to share the news, we began to unapologetically panic for the umpteenth time.

"Elevated pancreatic enzymes? What? This can't be happening. She did her time. She paid for the sins of her colon already. This has to be a joke."

"She is heading up to Rochester right now with Bill and we can help out with the girls."

Again.

Again, we all fulfilled our roles in helping them with whatever they needed. That had always been our job and we were more than happy to do it once more. But in the back of all of our heads, we were all scared and angry. Angry at the universe for tossing her yet another curve ball.

Bill and Danielle had to go through the ER department once more. And once more they had to wait awhile before she was given a room even in the ER department. When she was finally placed, the "room" was really the size of a closet with a curtain partition in the middle and on the other side was another patient.

Evening turned into night and they were visited by a doctor from the GI department who said they were unsure of what to do with her and thought that maybe the general surgeon on call could provide a different perspective. Her symptoms were leading them down the gallbladder path but this wasn't a textbook case so there was more than a shred of uncertainty with the diagnosis.

They waited some more in their tiny cavern of a room, both getting little or no sleep as the night wore on. At one point, when Bill had gone to the restroom, per the hospital's protocol, Danielle was approached by a social worker.

"Danielle, we just want to make sure you are safe at home?"

She tried not to chuckle because they were just doing their job but she was more than safe at home and was made even more grateful in that moment for her fabulous husband. She knew that there were women who did not have the same fortune as her and fell victim to the unthinkable.

"Yes, I am definitely safe at home. But I really appreciate you checking on me."

The morning dawned on them and they were *still* in the ER. She had lost yet another day in her life to the confines of a hospital. Up to this point, over the course of six years, she had occupied almost 45 days there; a month and a half of her life spent as a sick person. An experience most of us will never understand personally.

They were finally given some answers, though. The general surgeon arrived and decided it was most likely the gallbladder but they wouldn't officially know until they got in there to see for themselves. Based on the pain that she was still experiencing, she gave them the green light to open her up. She was then moved up to a real room for the remainder of that Saturday, after a full 24 hours down in the ER. The surgery was scheduled for first thing Sunday morning. She was relieved to have a plan but was not relieved of the intractable pain that was her new constant companion.

My mom and Steve picked me up very early on Sunday morning and we headed up to the hospital for the fourth time in 16 months. We were able to see her before surgery which allowed us to meet the very nice and seemingly competent surgeon. He reiterated to us that it seemed like her gallbladder was the culprit but that they would obviously know more once they could see it more clearly. We said our goodbyes and this time the goal kept everyone's emotions in check: get her feeling better.

We were told that if it was the gallbladder the procedure would last potentially an hour so back to the lobby we went. We got coffee. We read magazines. We tried to make each other laugh but an hour turned into two and then we began to get nervous. My mom and I pummeled Steve with questions since he is in an OR for the majority of his day. Thankfully, he is almost always even keeled and was not one bit nervous. He was gracious in mollifying our irrational worries when we heard the P.A. system start.

"Can the family of Danielle Eaton please come to the information desk?"

The front desk attendant called for Bill and we all headed for the desk. Since it was Sunday, they didn't update the public monitor screen like they do during the week so we didn't see her progress from one area to the next like we had before.

"Yes, uh huh. Okay. Wow. Well, good. Thank you, doctor."

"What did he say?" My mom and I impatiently said those words in unison as if he weren't going to tell us.

"They did remove her gallbladder. But he said that it wasn't too bad. However, it would have eventually needed to come out. They noticed something else. She also had something called an infarcted omentum and he believes that was the cause of all of her pain and symptoms."

"An infarcted o-what?" I inquired.

From watching Dr. Oz on Oprah many moons ago (during the good ol' days of afternoon TV), I suddenly remembered him showing her what an omentum was. It is an "apron-like" layer of fat that hangs down from our stomach and liver. In heavier-set people it gets quite large (that's what Dr. Oz was pointing out on the episode I watched) but we all have one. So, I did have a reference point for that part of the diagnosis but the "infarcted" part tripped me up.

All I could conjure up in my brain when hearing the word "infarcted" was Scut Farkus from the classic holiday film, *A Christmas Story*. *(Side note – I always thought it was Scott but thanks to the infinite wisdom of the Internet, I was corrected immediately.)* The famous narrated line from the movie played out in my head, "Scut Farkus staring out at us with his yellow eyes. He had yellow eyes! So, help me, God! Yellow eyes!"

I was snapped back to reality quickly thanks to Steve's medical explanation.

"Well, it isn't common but it just means that a piece of the omentum twists and twists on itself and eventually begins to die off because it isn't receiving a blood supply. When there is pain associated with it, it closely resembles the feeling you have with a Charlie horse. Here's another way to understand it, think of a plastic straw, if you bend it in half and start twisting it, you can no longer suck up fluid nor can you push anything out. In essence, that's what happens. If the omentum dies and becomes necrotic tissue, then you can have major problems. In Danielle's case, the infarction is probably tied to scar tissue she has from the various surgery points over the last year."

Phew!

We rejoiced. We had an answer and the problem was solved. Not just a little bit solved but 100% put-a-fork-in-it solved. We saw the doctor again as we visited

Danielle in the recovery room and he said something that he normally doesn't.

"I can honestly say with total certainty that this was her problem all along and she's going to feel worlds better, which is something I never tell my patients. The pain will be gone and she'll be just fine."

I wondered out loud about the pancreatic enzymes that we'd all been worried about and was told that could have been underlying gallbladder disease since she did have some basic symptoms. Another theory was that her body was reacting as if there was an infection, which could have accounted for the elevation. Sepsis was then discussed as a potential outcome if this hadn't been resolved. The infection could have made it to her bloodstream and she would have been in peril.

Say it with me…. again!

Not this time though. She was finally one step ahead.

Eventually they kicked us out of the recovery room and told us they would let us know when she was back upstairs and we could visit. We all took a collective deep breath and the seriousness of what could have been began to float away. We chatted and smiled and before long we were back in the elevator heading up to greet her. We happened to catch her being wheeled onto the floor and as she became more alert, the first thing she did was reach for her belly.

"The pain is gone. It doesn't hurt. It feels a lot better."

She smiled big and so did we.

Bill stayed with her that night while my mom, Steve, and I went home. We were exhausted but mostly thankful. She had dodged a bullet and was going to be okay.

The next morning her GI surgeon came to check on her. Danielle was secretly very glad to see her because she had felt validated with the general surgeon's findings. No one believed that what she had was anything other than a virus. Though it wasn't the GI doctor's fault for not knowing, Danielle was just happy they had the chance to talk about it.

"Danielle, this all makes sense now. But of all the things for you to have, this is incredibly rare. You are like the Jesus of colon surgeries – you've taken on every complication so other patients don't have to."

Amen sister.

For the first time in her journey of hospital stays, and on the monumental tenth time (she should have gotten a VIP punch card), she only had to stay for one night and then was discharged for good behavior. She was able to convalesce at home for a week and that's all she needed. The following Monday she put on her fancy dress shoes and headed back to work. She did not have a lot of sick time stored up thanks to the other surgeries but this post-op experience was different. She was assuredly getting better every day and did not have a single complication or setback. There has to be a first time for everything. Danielle just decided to wait until the end of the line to give that old saying some credence.

CHAPTER 12

I would love to tell you that her story of ER visits and bizarre auto-immune glitches ended with the infarcted omentum. But alas, it didn't.

She had one more unexpected trip to the ER in the fall of 2019 that had us all fearing the worst. She developed dreadful stomach pain and a fever and which led her to believe she was experiencing a blockage. We dug out our worry hats from the back of the closet and placed them on our heads with hope that this time would be different. My mom went to the hospital to provide support and called me on her way to provide the few details we had.

"For the love of God mom, please let this be something normal or something common and treatable. I don't believe she could go through something traumatic and painful once more," I emphatically stated.

The truth is that she could have gone through it again because Danielle is one tough cannoli. Thankfully, though, she didn't have to. The heavens were shining down on her that day and allowed it to just be a run-of-the-mill stomach virus (this was pre-COVID-19 here in the United States, thus, we were okay with it just being a virus of unknown origin). Apparently, viruses really can settle in funny places and she happened to have caught one that started as a cold and migrated south for the winter, into her belly. She bounced back after a few days and we took off our worry hats.

And then we burned those suckers.

Unfortunately, the heavens *did* afford Danielle the pleasure of having to deal with two other auto-immune malfunctions in 2019 and 2020: alopecia and external cervical root reabsorption. Both of which are more fun than a barrel of monkeys.

Alopecia is essentially baldness where hair normally grows. For Danielle, an attractive gal who has to dress up for work every day, her alopecia appeared in early 2019 and was located the top of her head for the world to see. If she parted her hair a certain way or wore a headband, she was able to disguise the patches with no hair. Fun factoid on the causes of alopecia, as defined by Google:

"Current evidence suggest that alopecia is caused by an abnormality in the immune system that damages hair follicles. This particular abnormality leads to autoimmunity, a misguided immune system that tends to attack its own body. As a result, the immune system attacks particular tissues of the body."

Misguided is right. We now know that Danielle's immune system is like Cinderella's awful step-sisters. It seems narrowly focused on causing harm and strife whenever and wherever it can. If only we could give it a hug and show it some empathy and love.

Thankfully, alopecia is somewhat common and the treatment involved steroid drops directly onto the affected areas to help spur her follicles to regrow. Sometimes it doesn't work but in Danielle's case, although it took many months, it did. She has regrown her hair and doesn't have to hide specific parts of her head any more.

Treating external cervical root reabsorption was not quite as easy and as a diagnosis, it is not as common. A show of hands please for all of you who have heard of it before?

Anyone?

Bueller?

In a nutshell, her body was attacking her own tooth, which caused it to slowly break away from her gumline. If this helps you understand how uncommon it is, when you type it into Google, the results are all verbose dental or medical journal articles. There isn't a basic description or definition that magically appears like you'd see when searching a more popular issue like hiccups or the flu.

The reason this occurs is debatable to some degree but her dentist felt that her wonky immune system could be at fault. It can be caused by trauma and though Danielle did not have any direct trauma to the affected tooth at the time it needed to be repaired, she did have a root canal many years before on that same tooth. Technically, it was dead already which is how she knew something was off, the area around the tooth started to feel odd after Christmas in 2018. It seemed irritated and the tooth itself began to feel wiggly. She made an appointment during her winter break from school and was not prepared for the diagnosis or the treatment plan. When her dentist explained what would happen over the coming months, six to nine to be exact, he had a long face.

Step one was to take an impression of her tooth so

they could fabricate a new one to put in its place once the bad tooth was removed. Step two occurred a few weeks later, and centered on the extraction. With forceps in hand, the dentist was able to pull it out entirely without any complications. He did have to use three sutures to allow her gums to heal back together. In the interim, she was fitted with a prosthetic tooth, attached to a retainer that was not very comfortable. At first, she committed to herself that no one would see her toothless, especially Bill. But because it did not fit perfectly in her mouth, she allowed us all to see her sans a front tooth on the second day. It gave us all a good laugh to see the gaping hole where there should be a tooth but she quickly shed any vanity hurdles that were initially in the way. Having a tube come out of her rear end, losing her hair in noticeable places, and then to become toothless, gave her a tangible sense of humility.

Step three, occurred five weeks later and was not a long appointment. Because her gums had healed over the spot where her original tooth was, they needed to cut the membrane to make a space for a metal cap that would hold the new tooth in place. "Cut" and "membrane" don't sound pleasing to the ear but she managed it really well and kept looking ahead.

Step four, which happened four months later in June of 2019, was the penultimate step and would give her the metal cap. The dentist had to drill a titanium rod into her jaw, which would eventually attach to the tooth. They gave her Novocain to numb the pain but the feeling was still disturbing for her. She felt as if they were drilling directly into her skull. Her dentist was wonderful throughout but it was still a long, arduous process that left her pretty exhausted by the day's end. She rebounded well and kept her focus on the end game: a new tooth that wouldn't spontaneously detach from her mouth.

A few weeks later, step five commenced. Her brand-new zirconia tooth found its home in her mouth. Because the new tooth is front and center of her smile, it is noticeable if you look closely and she smiles wide. To her, the imperfection the new tooth poses is a-okay. She could have gotten veneers and she could have gotten plastic surgery to remove the scars on her stomach yet she opted to keep her battle wounds as personal proof that she overcame an ordeal that felt insurmountable to her.

The great news about her new tooth was its timing. It was put in just before their big trip out west in late July of 2019. This excursion took a full two years to plan and execute and seemed like the real finish line for Danielle's marathon-long journey with auto-immune diseases. She had figuratively climbed a mountain and yearned to do it in person; to underscore the fact that she was no longer a "sick" woman living a muted life.

The seed for the trip was planted in the summer of 2017 when Danielle was recovering from surgery number three. She pulled an empty envelope from her desk and began to slowly sock money away for their planes, trains and automobiles adventure. Horace Greeley's homesteader advice, "Go West," reverberated in her head as she pitched the idea to Bill. Initially their goal was to take the kids to see the majestic Grand Canyon but that evolved into a multi-state extravaganza, which then came to include Death Valley, Yosemite, and San Francisco.

Over the course of the two-year planning period, Bill and Danielle made Thursday nights their special time devoted to hammering out the logistics of their itinerary. They would let Domino's make them dinner, pour themselves a cocktail, and sit before their computer making decisions on what to do and where to stay. It gave them great excitement to virtually explore the National Parks that they would eventually experience in person. Sometimes they would get so wrapped up in the fun of formulating their trip of a lifetime, they would forget to stop and eat. One night both Danielle and Bill were on their phones with various hotels, for an extended period of time, causing dinner to be pushed back. For two hungry, growing girls, this was completely unacceptable. So, Lily and May took matters into their own hands and slipped a napkin in front of Danielle that read, "When is dinner?" It made Danielle giggle and brought her back to reality. It was easy to get lost in the exciting details of what she had worked so hard to attain.

Once the trip was finalized it had blossomed into a full two-week tour of the West Coast. The first leg of the trip took them to the Grand Canyon and it was complete with a strenuous five-hour hike, in 95-degree heat, with the desert sun pouring down over them. Poor May wilted towards the end but she and Danielle took it slow and steady and were able to finish the trek. The hike was brutal on all of their legs but they managed it successfully just as the canyon's burnt sienna hues became more pronounced as the sun lowered in the sky. A marvelous vantage point that left them feeling tremendously thankful. They all took well-deserved naps once they were back at their hotel and then treated themselves to a delicious steak dinner to replenish their stores.

Next, they headed to the gorgeous but arid Death

Valley. Their resort, The Oasis, was charming and could have been the backdrop of a picture show set in the Golden Age of film. The temperatures were also cinema-worthy. When they arrived to their "casita," a little cottage on the property, at 1:00 in the morning, it was a balmy 101 degrees. Off in the distance, they could hear the unforgettable and disturbing sounds of cackling coyotes. The highest temperature they experienced was 118 degrees at 11:00 in the morning the next day. Yet again, the heat did not sit well with fair-skinned May, so she had to limit her time outside while she was there. For all of them, though, their time outside was spent in short bursts. For example, they visited sand dunes nearby (where Star Wars' Episodes IV and VI were filmed) and could only be outside of the car for a total of 15 minutes. They also toured the lowest spot in North America, Badwater Basin, which sits 282 feet below sea level. Danielle could only describe it as "scorched earth." They appreciated the unique landscape even though it felt like they were strolling on the bottom of the ocean without water because it was dry, salt-crusted land. They finished their time in Death Valley by eating dinner at The Last Kind Word Saloon. A fitting name for a spot isolated in the middle of the fiery desert.

Yosemite was next on the agenda and the car ride to get there was equal parts exhilarating and terrifying. On their way out of Death Valley, Danielle offered to give Bill a driving break and thought the scenic ascent into the park would be the perfect time. She was not prepared for the dangerous cliffs through mountainous terrain, the hairpin turns she had to navigate with the kids in the backseat, and the unwanted fear that crept into the back of her throat. She was able to channel her inner Mario

Andretti, however, and was able to white knuckle her way through the dangerous course. By the time they reached Yosemite, Bill was driving and it felt like they had arrived at Shangri-La.

Yosemite is one of the bigger parks in the National Park system and everything about their time there was a dream come true. The resort, Rush Creek Lodge, and its amenities, were luxurious. All of the buildings were adorned with stone and cedar and there was an emphasis on outdoor activities (i.e., outdoor grills, beautiful pools, hot tubs, playgrounds). Their room faced the mountains with gorgeous panoramas of the mountain range. It was everything their two years of planning could provide. While in the park, they visited Glacier Point overlook, the infamous granite monolith El Capitan, and Half Dome, also a massive granite rock formation. They were also lucky enough to tour through a forest of giant sequoia trees and swim in the frosty Merced River, which was only 50 degrees on the day they waded in. For Danielle, the highlight of their time at Yosemite occurred entirely thanks to her "new" parts.

She needed to use the restroom and had to meander down from the waterfall area where they were to find the bathroom. As she neared her destination, she noticed the large creatures she had been hoping to spot the whole time they were there, a gorgeous mama bear and her small furry cub. A park ranger was nearby keeping park guests safe and informed but allowed the onlookers to get close enough to admire the beauty of seeing these wild animals in person. Danielle was able to call Bill and the kids and they quickly headed down to meet her. They spent about two hours stalking the bears before they decided to move on. She was ecstatic though having fulfilled her dream of seeing bears at Yosemite. It wouldn't have occurred if she didn't need to frequent the bathroom.

The last leg of their adventure had them putting away their hiking boots and grabbing their sweatshirts as they headed even further west for foggy San Francisco. On their way, they drove through almond and walnut groves and took in the beauty of California farmlands. It reminded Danielle of the bountiful Tuscan countryside she had enjoyed years before. They were only in San Fran for two days and nights but they packed a lot of sightseeing in their time there. They saw all of the traditional touristy hot spots via a retro Volkswagen bus ride called the Love at Night tour. They also visited Fisherman's Wharf and dined on clam chowder, saw the highlights and felt the warmth of Sausalito, and biked across the Golden Gate Bridge. They even had time to take a ferry over to the infamous Alcatraz Prison and nearby Angel Island before taking a red eye flight home.

They were tired and bleary-eyed but once they were back, they reveled in the whirlwind tour of breathtaking locations they were lucky enough to have just seen. The prior two summers had been spent with doctors and involved uncomfortable hospital beds and more IVs than they could count. This trip, however, was the exact opposite. It was not depressing. It did not include bad news. And it did not require surgical intervention. It did what all good vacations are supposed to do and then some. It provided a respite from her former life and a glimpse into what the future would hold.

Yes, Danielle and Bill were happy to have a fresh

start. Her new, healthy body allowed them to look ahead to 2020 and beyond with hope in their eyes and a longing in their hearts for new adventures.

Oh, and they couldn't wait to buy toilet paper on the black market and to start wiping down their groceries before putting them away.

Just kidding about the last part!

But what an interesting book that will make.

EPILOGUE

If you are not a UC survivor, you should take a minute and repeat after me.

"Thank you, colon."

Because as you've just read, it can rob you of a normal life. I'm hopeful, though, that you will take this story and not focus on the bloody poop I discussed (it *still* feels embarrassing and naughty to type those words even as I wrap this up) but rather hone in on all of the moments where resilience won. As humans going through life, we are all tested in a myriad of ways – mentally, physically, and spiritually. And that is what Danielle's story really encompasses: the ability for a person, who was arguably dealt a bad hand, to rise above the sorrow that temporarily permeated her life and push on.

In the fall of 2019, she saw her beloved PCP for her annual physical and for the first time in eleven years, her blood work was perfect. Her doctor was so taken with her progress that even he, a tremendously busy man, took the time to walk down memory lane with her. They went over the triumphs and travails of adapting to life with UC and ultimately succumbing to it. But they were able to smile at the notion that she'd come to the other side and would be able to live a mostly-normal life going forward. She was given a second chance and she knew it.

And because she had the presence of mind to

understand what could have been versus what really was, at Christmas time in 2019, she decided to send her GI surgeon a Christmas card which featured a family picture from their family vacation out West. It's an enviable snapshot of the four of them with Yosemite National Park in the background on the front of the card, and the Grand Canyon on the back. Along with the card, she sent her a more detailed letter. In the note she included her true feelings for the gift that the surgeon had given her. In so many words, this is what Danielle communicated:

"I wouldn't have been able to do this hike and take this trip without you. It took three surgeries, and many side effects later but because of your work, I was able to hike down the mountain in Yosemite – five total miles with many switchbacks. I was also able to do a six-mile hike in the Grand Canyon. And don't worry, I was good about staying hydrated and drinking my Gatorade. But, I was also able to enjoy a glass of wine or two! Overall, I was able to accomplish something wonderful that I wouldn't have been able to otherwise. You have my permission to show this card to your patients who may be feeling hopeless so they know there is light at the end of the tunnel."

She mailed it off and didn't think about the card again until her annual checkup and colonoscopy with her surgeon in the summer of 2020. When they were going over the results (which were normal!) Danielle asked her surgeon if she had received the card.

"Yes! Oh my goodness. Thank you for sending it. I can't tell you how many patients I've shown this to. The card stays with me but it bounces back and forth between my office and the hospital."

Because the surgeon was in scrubs, she didn't

reach in her very nice purse to dig it out but she was equally as grateful to have it in her possession. Danielle smiled from ear to ear knowing that her life, captured in a card, was being shared to help others.

For the most part, 2020 was kind to Danielle's body. Despite the swirling pandemic around her, she was able to skate through the year having to only deal with one unpleasant auto-immune problem: thrush.

This lovely disorder is a tough one to describe in PG terms. I apologize but you'll need to brace yourself for a few unpleasant words. Thrush is the condition where a yeast-like fungus overgrows in one's mouth and throat. In other words, it's a yeast infection. Unsurprisingly, Google says that it's a common occurrence for babies, people with immune deficiencies (ahem, Danielle Eaton), and folks who use oral steroid sprays to control asthma.

She didn't know what it was at first and attributed her symptoms to heartburn. She called her PCP and he prescribed typical acid reflux medicine that seemed to help somewhat. When it didn't go away her GI doctor was brought into the mix and he scheduled her for an EGD. EGD stands for the following super long spelling bee word: esophagogastroduodenoscopy. An EGD is a procedure that looks at the upper portion of a person's GI tract. Essentially, it's like a colonoscopy for your esophagus and stomach. She had to be anesthetized for the process and was a nervous wreck. Her mind immediately went to Crohn's. She was fearful that the pain and burning she experienced were ulcers in her throat. What the doctor found, though, were white spots indicative of a yeast infection. All she needed was a prescription for Nystatin, a medication that fights off infections such as these and thankfully, it worked like a charm. She found total relief after a week.

As we all watched the horrors of COVID-19 from March through the fall, Danielle remained healthy. She wore her mask, played by the rules, and even got her flu shot early. She thought by getting her shot she was helping her body but in reality, the act of testing her immune system caused thrush to develop once more. It started with heartburn and before she realized what was happening, her tongue became fuzzy and covered in those same white lesions.

In March it seemed as if the thrush were a fluke. Seven months later and post-flu shot, it was not a coincidence. Her immune system was at fault. Her response to coming down with it again, was typical for Danielle and her positivity.

"Well, the remedy doesn't involve any tubes or surgery so I will be just fine. It could be a lot worse."

Yes, it sure could and she knows it because she lived it.

Danielle's tale was unique to her but the themes running throughout it and the strength she had to find within herself to keep going are universal. That sentiment was the impetus of this book and our hope for getting it into the hands of people who need it. In a time of UC crisis and despair, there is a palpable power in knowing that others in a similar situation were able to successfully navigate the poop-related path put before them. It might not always be an easy path but if you have a map or a guide, such as this book, you can traverse it with less fear and less anxiety.

And hopefully less toilet paper.

If you have a question or a concern about your way forward as a UC superhero, email us at UCquestion@gmail.com. We are not doctors, nurses, or psychologists. We cannot diagnose, treat or weigh in on your symptoms. If you are seeking medical or therapeutic advice, please call your physician, or Dr. Phil. However, we *can* speak about our experiences as the patient and the patient's cheerleader. Danielle can share details about her journey, what worked for her, and what did not. And I can speak to being a helpless bystander. Because sometimes all you need is a kindred spirit to validate what you are feeling and that what you are going through is *really* hard.

And someone who you can talk poop with.

Be well and thank you for choosing her story.

IMAGES

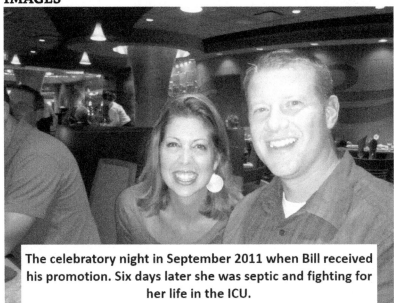

The celebratory night in September 2011 when Bill received his promotion. Six days later she was septic and fighting for her life in the ICU.

Sigmoidoscopy Exam Images

Patient:	Danielle Eaton	**Attending Physician:**
Patient ID:	MRN-0379869	**Referring Physician:**
Exam Date:	10/01/2011	

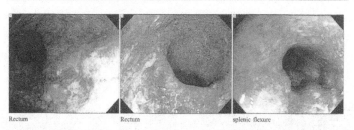

Rectum   Rectum   splenic flexure

Danielle's first colonoscopy imagery, October 2011. It was a terrible mess inside her large colon.

Colonoscopy Exam Images

Patient: danielle eaton   Attending Physician:
Patient ID: MRN-h001070146   Referring Physician:
Exam Date: 11/21/2011

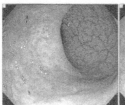 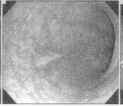 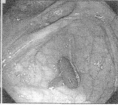

rectum   sigmoid

Taken one month after being in the ICU. She was making great strides towards remission, November 2011.

Patient:	danielle eaton		Attending Physician:
Patient ID:	MRN-0379869		Referring Physician:
Exam Date:	04/02/2012		

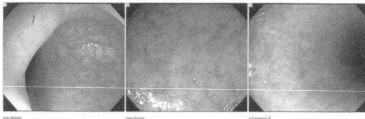

rectum   rectum   sigmoid

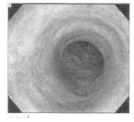

This is what a normal colon looks like and in April of 2012, it meant remission for Danielle.

Sigmoidoscopy Exam Images

Patient:	Danielle Eaton	Attending Physician:
Patient ID:	MRN-0379869	Referring Physician:
Exam Date:	03/10/2014	

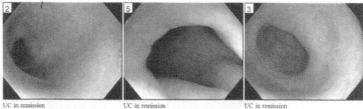

UC in remission   UC in remission   UC in remission

UC in remission   UC in remission

Still looking good two years later in March 2014.

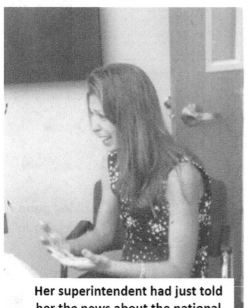

Her superintendent had just told her the news about the national teacher contest when this was snapped, May 2015.

Sigmoidoscopy Exam Images

Patient: Danielle Eaton   Attending Physician:
Patient ID: MRN-0379869   Referring Physician:
Exam Date: 03/24/2016

1 -rectum   2 -rectum

uc   4 -rectum

This was done a month after BillFest and showed the first signs of trouble looming, March 2016.

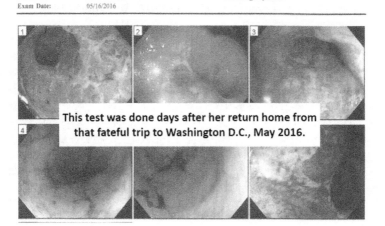

Sigmoidoscopy Exam Images

Patient:	Danielle Eaton	Attending Physician:
Patient ID:	MRN-0379869	Referring Physician:
Exam Date:	05/16/2016	

This test was done days after her return home from that fateful trip to Washington D.C., May 2016.

Sigmoidoscopy Exam Images

Patient:	Danielle Eaton	Attending Physician:
Patient ID:	MRN-0379869	Referring Physician:
Exam Date:	06/29/2016	

COLITIS   COLITIS   COLITIS

COLITIS

And the pièce de résistance, taken during her second hospital stay that summer, the end of June 2016.

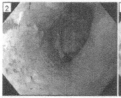
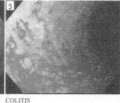
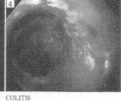

This series of pictures from her hospital stay related to the last colonoscopy images (June 2016) can be captioned as follows...

"I resemble a horse."   "I heart IV fluids."   "Steroids, oh sweet steroids."

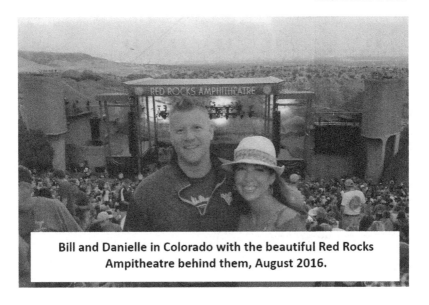

Bill and Danielle in Colorado with the beautiful Red Rocks Ampitheatre behind them, August 2016.

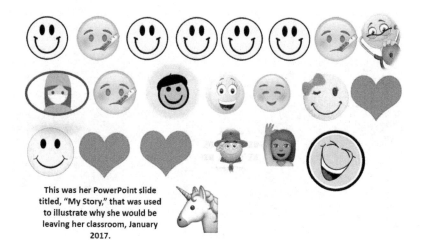

This was her PowerPoint slide titled, "My Story," that was used to illustrate why she would be leaving her classroom, January 2017.

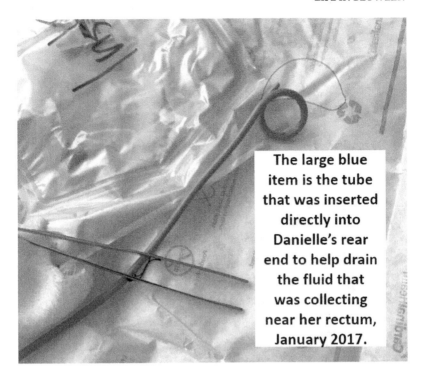

The large blue item is the tube that was inserted directly into Danielle's rear end to help drain the fluid that was collecting near her rectum, January 2017.

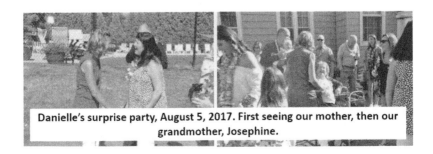

Danielle's surprise party, August 5, 2017. First seeing our mother, then our grandmother, Josephine.

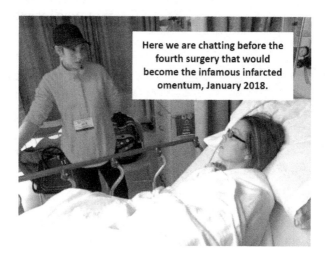

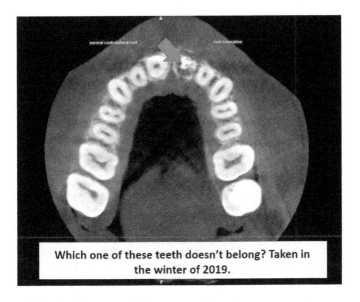

Which one of these teeth doesn't belong? Taken in the winter of 2019.

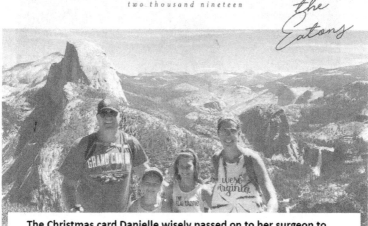

The Christmas card Danielle wisely passed on to her surgeon to inspire others. The picture was taken in August 2019.

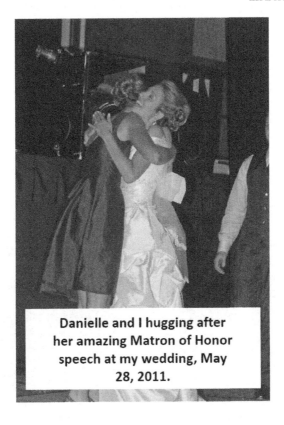

Danielle and I hugging after her amazing Matron of Honor speech at my wedding, May 28, 2011.

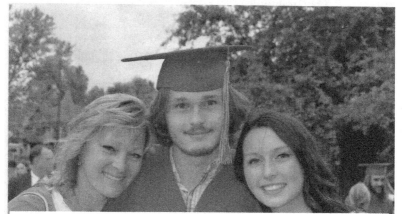

Our wonderful step-mom Shayne, our "little" brother Andrea, and our little sister Victoria at Andrea's high school graduation, June 2018.

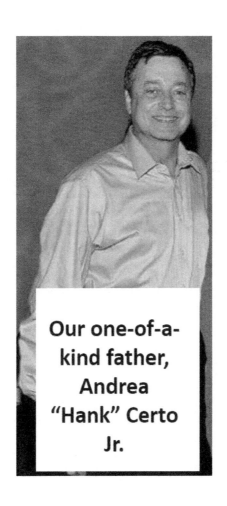

Our one-of-a-
kind father,
Andrea
"Hank" Certo
Jr.

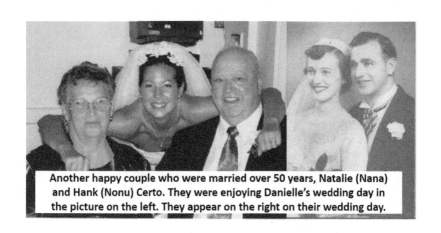

Another happy couple who were married over 50 years, Natalie (Nana) and Hank (Nonu) Certo. They were enjoying Danielle's wedding day in the picture on the left. They appear on the right on their wedding day.

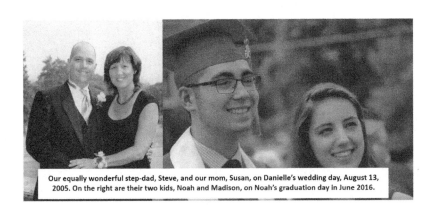

Our equally wonderful step-dad, Steve, and our mom, Susan, on Danielle's wedding day, August 13, 2005. On the right are their two kids, Noah and Madison, on Noah's graduation day in June 2016.

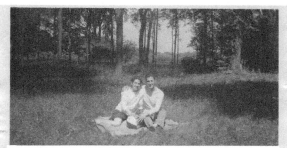

Our other grandparents, Josephine and Philip
Catanese, in an undated picture.

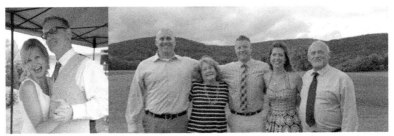

Danielle's fantastic in-laws, the Eatons. From left to right, Bill's sister Erica and her husband Rudy, Bill's younger brother, Gregory, his mother, Rhonda, Bill, Danielle, and big Gregg, Bill's father.

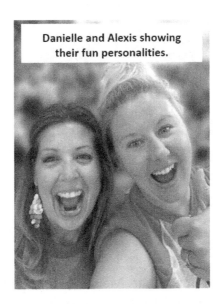

Danielle and Alexis showing their fun personalities.

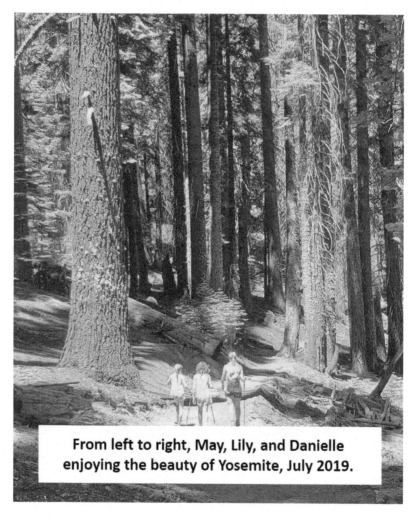

From left to right, May, Lily, and Danielle enjoying the beauty of Yosemite, July 2019.

ACKNOWLEDGEMENT

Writing this book was harder than I thought and yet, equally as satisfying. It had always been a goal of mine to formally tell a good literary story and although Danielle's story wasn't always "good," it had a happy ending that I was thrilled to share. My gratitude for her willingness to spend time with me while I asked very detailed questions about her painful past, is incalculable. I'm reminded on a daily basis of how thankful I am that she survived and that we can continue being sisters and friends.

To the other cast of characters in our lives that weave in and out of the story, I appreciate your patience and time. Both for reading rough drafts and for also answering my litany of questions. Bill, Mom, Steve, Madison, Noah, Dad, Shayne, Victoria, Andrea. Though your parts in the book may not be as pronounced, collectively, your role in helping her heal and providing support during her bleakest times, cannot be quantified. She and I were blessed to be born into a wonderful, loving family. T'amo.

If she were writing this acknowledgement, I know that she'd like to recognize Bill's fantastic family. His parents and siblings, Gregg, Rhonda, Erica and Gregory, lived this process with them as well and helped to carry them through to the other side.

Our extended families, on both our mom and dad's

sides, epitomize what big, Italian (and part Polish) famiglias are supposed to be: caring, thoughtful, and present. Our grandparents, aunts, uncles, and cousins, were there when she needed them and when they couldn't be there physically, they were there in spirit. To the Certos and Cataneses, another big T'amo from the both of us.

Alexis Roesser, Danielle's teaching best friend in crime, could also be considered a family member and should be recognized for her compassion and unending encouragement for Danielle. But mostly for her humor and wit. She's tremendously funny and was a tremendous friend throughout the entire ordeal.

To the people who helped me bring this Word document to a printed book, I am eternally grateful: Ryan McCarthy, Jessica Ongko, Dr. Steve Carlson, Diana McElfresh, Julie Morton, and Brad Gross. Grazie mille. Without your professional attributes and skills, it would have remained a Word document on my laptop. I will bake you free cupcakes for life. I promise.

Lastly, to my three favorite people, Sadie, Sawyer, and Mike, who saw me run to my desk when an idea struck me or when I had to sneak in time for corrections, I am beyond appreciative that you were patient. Thank you for allowing me to dive so deep into something that I am now able to share with the world.

ABOUT THE AUTHOR

Natalie Smith

Natalie Smith received her bachelor's degree in Mass Communications and has a master's degree in Conflict Resolution. She began her career in mediation as a Florida Supreme Court Certified Mediator in 2008 and has taught online classes and workshops for over ten years. She has a passion for books and writing as well as baking fancy cakes. She lives in Western New York with 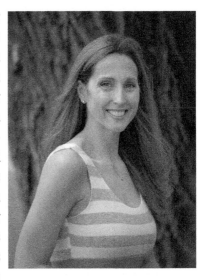 her husband Mike and her kids, Sadie and Sawyer.

Made in the USA
Middletown, DE
24 July 2021